Speech Anxiety and Stuttering

101 essential questions and answers

By Olga Bednarski BA (Hons), MSc Psych.
and *the Crew*

Holistic Wellness Publishing, Liverpool 2025

Holistic Wellbeing Publishing, Liverpool 2025

Cover design by Jane Cornwell

Table of Contents

Disclaimer: This book is dedicated to addressing psychological speech anxiety (stuttering) in adults. The book and the tools it offers are NOT suitable for developmental stuttering in children. If you believe your stuttering is caused by organic trauma to the speech apparatus, cranial damage, shell shock, stroke or a mechanically inflicted trauma to the breathing organs or brain, please seek professional medical advice and guidance.

The methodology and tools offered in this book do not represent a fast resolution, often referred to as a 'magic pill', nor are they an instant miraculous cure. The process of dissolving stuttering in adults requires time, dedication and the consistent application of techniques over a minimum period of six months.

Whether you choose to use the techniques offered in this book or not, the author is not responsible for any consequences resulting from your decisions. Whatever you decide to do with the information provided is entirely at your discretion, and you assume full responsibility for the outcomes.

'Everything is shown up by being exposed to the light. And whatever is exposed to the light itself becomes light.'

— Saint Paul

'Stuttering is not just a challenge; it's a doorway to something much greater within each individual. The challenge is the door to discovering who you truly are!'

— Olga Bednarski

'In my work, I sometimes encounter people who stutter who are difficult to work with – there are resistance, misconceptions and deep-seated beliefs about stuttering being an incurable disease, a myth fed to people for hundreds of years. However, when I view my mission as raising a child – with all its occasional tantrums, frustrations and moments of exhaustion – I am reminded of the immense joy that comes from watching that child grow and thrive. It's not an easy job, but in the grand scheme of things, it is absolutely worth it.'

— Olga Bednarski

'With Olga's approach, stuttering is under arrest – without the right for parole!'

— YouTube Channel subscriber

To all the incredible souls I have met along this journey of understanding speech anxiety (aka stuttering).

Thank you for your questions, your comments, your criticism and for challenging me in ways that shaped and deepened my understanding. Each of you has been a teacher, offering me a piece of the puzzle, urging me to look deeper for answers and inspiring me to refine my ideas and explanations.

Your courage, curiosity and contributions have been invaluable, and I hold immense gratitude in my heart. You have helped bring this unique approach to life, and for that I am forever thankful.

This book is my gift to you all.

With all my love,

Olga

Introduction

The way you perceive a problem or task, and the depth of your understanding, shapes your entire approach to solving it. This includes whether you choose to address it or let it be, the strategies and tools you employ, how you implement those strategies and the timeline you establish for resolving the issue or completing the task.

Let's consider a simple example. Imagine you want to hang a picture on a wooden wall. You understand what's required, and with the right tools in hand, you anticipate it will take just a few minutes. Armed with a hammer and a nail, you drive the nail into the wall, securing it firmly. Once the nail is in place, you hang the picture – a quick, straightforward and satisfying process.

Now, let's shift the scenario slightly. Imagine that the wall isn't made of wood but concrete. Would you approach the task in the same way? Likely not. Using the same tools and method wouldn't work, and the task would remain incomplete. Instead, you'd need to adapt – choosing a drill instead of a hammer and screws rather than nails. With the right understanding and tools, you'd once again achieve your goal, this time with a sense of ingenuity and perseverance.

The skilled and experienced handyman knows exactly which tools and strategies to choose to align with the specific task at hand. Without this understanding, failure is inevitable. You cannot blame the wall for being made of concrete, nor can you fault the hammer for being unsuitable for the job, or the nail for not penetrating the surface. The only failure lies in not thoughtfully assessing the task, evaluating its requirements and selecting the right tools to complete it effectively.

Addressing speech anxiety or stuttering is no different.[1] It, too, is a task – one that requires a deep and compassionate understanding of the challenge you face. To overcome it, you must carefully analyse how your stuttering functions and choose a tailored set of tools to address each facet of this intricate issue – mental, emotional and physical. By doing so, you set yourself

[1] Even though stuttering, as a symptom, originates from anxiety, the terms stuttering and speech anxiety are used interchangeably throughout this book and have the same meaning.

firmly on the path towards your ultimate goal: freedom from irrational social fears, anxiety and panic. This thoughtful approach opens the door to effortless, enjoyable interactions with others and grants you the confidence to engage fully with the world around you.

Once you truly understand what you are dealing with and become consciously aware of the inner workings of stuttering, the path forward becomes clearer. The problem that has weighed so heavily on you for years – even decades – begins to loosen its grip on your emotional, social, personal and professional life, as well as your physical well-being. As your understanding deepens and you gain greater conscious control, your once-crippling anxiety starts to fade, creating space for clarity and peace of mind.

This newfound clarity is a gift – it makes room for all the meaningful aspects of life that may have once seemed out of reach. Relationships, career opportunities, new acquaintances, fresh experiences – all these possibilities come into view. When you identify and confront the forces that have been holding you back, you are no longer at the mercy of a 'mysterious condition' or an unpredictable force. Instead, you reclaim your power, and with it the ability to chart a new trajectory, free from fear.

Too often, I meet individuals who stutter yet remain unaware of the deeper nature of their verbal struggles. This is profoundly heart-wrenching. Many have spent years in traditional speech therapy, where the focus is almost entirely on the mechanical aspects of speech. While well-intentioned, this narrow approach neglects the critical psychological components of speech anxiety. As a result, people often find themselves trapped – unable to break free from the emotional chains of anxiety or achieve lasting progress.

Even those who manage to experience some improvement frequently relapse within a short time. Without the right tools to self-regulate, they become overly reliant on coaches or therapists to stabilize their emotions and regain their balance. This dependency robs them of the ability to independently restore emotional equilibrium, find inner peace and express themselves fluently.

After more than 14 years of personal and professional experience, my heartfelt conviction is this: people who stutter (PWS) need education far more than they need a 'cure'. The staggering array of existing theories – often conflicting, convoluted and attempting to 'debunk the myth of stuttering' – highlights a glaring reality. As of today (December 2024), there is no clear consensus or universally accepted understanding of stuttering. Consequently, there is also no widely effective or adaptable solution to empower individuals to shed the victim mentality and embrace the tools they need to achieve their dreams.

Too often, I see people facing the immovable 'concrete wall' of misinformation and misunderstanding. They are encouraged to keep trying, yet without the right approach or insight, they're essentially attempting to 'drive a nail into a concrete wall with a hammer'. Predictably, these misguided efforts lead to failure. For those with severe stuttering, repeated failures carve a painful path towards despair, chronic disease, hopelessness, feelings of inferiority, isolation and often secondary mental health challenges.

The majority of PWS are misinformed and lack a clear understanding of themselves and the true nature of their predicament. They persistently rely on tools and strategies that are entirely unsuitable for the task at hand. Again and again, they attempt the same ineffective approach – trying to drive that metaphorical nail into concrete – and each time they're left feeling frustrated and defeated. This endless cycle of trial and error paves the way for even more convoluted theories and so-called 'cures', which often mislead and disappoint. Consider extreme measures like injecting Botox into the thoracic muscles to prevent glottal spasms – a solution that promises much but delivers little.

The core reason so many people struggle is that they rely on methods shaped by societal expectations and widespread misconceptions about stuttering. These methods fail to address the actual challenges they face. In contrast, those who achieve meaningful improvement – or even complete freedom from stuttering – are not merely fortunate. They have taken a fundamentally different approach. They have chosen to question conventional wisdom, set aside traditional views on stuttering and explore alternative paths to 'solve the riddle' that so many still deem unsolvable.

'Exclude yourself from the rule! Step away from the statistics, and you will achieve heights that once seemed impossible for someone like you.'

— Olga Bednarski, author of *The Anatomy of Stuttering*

The key to unlocking the door to freedom lies in changing how you view the problem. This truth applies to any challenge – not just stuttering. New knowledge and solutions already exist, waiting for those willing to open their eyes and hearts. The door is unlocked; it's up to you to step through.

It's time for more people to pull back the curtain on outdated, widely accepted, yet often misinformed theories. It's time to look beyond stuttering, grasp the essence of the problem and embrace strategies that are not only effective but also transformative. These approaches, while perhaps not institutionalized or mainstream within traditional speech pathology, hold the potential to truly address the challenge at its core.

The goal of this book is twofold: to provide much-needed education – 'knowledge therapy' – to PWS worldwide, empowering them to face themselves with honesty and compassion, and to guide them out of the maze of theoretical complexity. It seeks to place them firmly on a path towards a life where communication no longer stirs anxiety but instead brings joy, excitement, meaning and connection.

Simply talking about fluency, reading books, engaging in theoretical debates or watching instructional videos on how to control blocking will never be enough. While these resources can offer valuable guidance, information alone is not sufficient. To eliminate anxiety and fear and achieve lasting fluency, knowledge must be applied, internalized and woven into daily life. It must become a lived, embodied experience – transforming your thoughts, feelings, emotions, attitudes, behaviours and responses to the everyday moments when you speak.

Fluency is a holistic concept as well as a state of being (**a mindset**) that reaches far beyond speech. It encompasses the inner dynamics of the individual – their thoughts, emotions and sense of self. Through real-life examples, my goal is to help PWS recognize how they unconsciously create experiences of disfluency, struggle and anxiety. With care and compassion, I hope to gently guide them towards greater self-awareness and the conscious cultivation of a lived experience of fluency and fluidity in their everyday lives.

Why this book?

This book is intended to be a guiding light for those still lost in the darkness of complexity, helping them to finally see the path and take their first steps forward. It seeks to help readers cross the bridge – from darkness to light, from ignorance to understanding and from self-judgment to self-compassion.

Who Is This Book For?

This book is for individuals who stutter and for therapists who, despite the dominant 'conclusive' scientific and medical narrative framing stuttering as 'an incurable genetic condition', remain open to the possibility that there is more to stuttering than meets the eye. It is for those willing to explore beyond surface-level explanations, equipping themselves with an alternative and holistic understanding of the issue – one that does not isolate speech from the individual but instead embraces the often-overlooked dynamics of the human inner world, including thoughts, emotions and feelings.

This book introduces a flexible, comprehensive and deeply holistic approach to addressing and dissolving the problem – an approach that views fluency as an integral part of the whole person, rather than merely a function of speech.

I understand that some of you may already practise positive thinking and strive to accept your stuttering as an inseparable and unavoidable part of who you are. However, it's just as important to be sincere and honest with yourself. If you're engaging in positive thinking while continuing to struggle daily with anxiety, fear, panic, denial, shame and guilt – before, during and after social interactions – then true acceptance may still be out of reach.

If you avoid certain situations or turn down valuable opportunities out of fear of exposing your stutter, feel inferior to fluent speakers or punish yourself after perceived 'failures', then you're not fully accepting your condition. Instead, you may be clinging to a façade, one that denies you the peace, freedom and authenticity you deserve.

Recognizing this truth is essential – not to blame or criticize yourself, but to inspire a thoughtful re-evaluation of your approach to self-understanding, the challenges you face and the methods you currently use to address them. Instead, consider embracing effective, natural, simple and even enjoyable tools and practices that can help dissolve most, if not all, of your inner conflicts and irrational fears. These methods have the potential to improve your emotional well-being and foster genuine self-acceptance.

When you reach this stage, the need for 'forced' or socially conditioned acceptance ('*my community says it's the right thing to do*') will naturally fade away. In its place, you'll find a newfound mental freedom – space for greater creativity, restful sleep, new opportunities, meaningful relationships and the pursuit of dreams you may have once deemed impossible or forbidden.

If, despite conflicting scientific claims, someone somewhere has overcome stuttering – transforming their life from severe daily anxiety and blocking into one of harmony, inner peace, balance and freedom – then I want you to know this: you can do it too.

A gentle reminder: the information in this book will only help if you choose to apply it. By turning theoretical knowledge into practical wisdom and lived experience, you can create lasting change. It's then that you'll begin to experience a profound and life-changing transformation.

Remember, no single method, course, technique or seminar can instantly bring about permanent healing, reshape your mindset or transform your personality forever. Like anything truly worthwhile in life, inner transformation takes time, dedication and consistent application to fully integrate into your being – to become a natural and essential part of your 'updated' self. Meaningful change cannot happen overnight.

For many of you, your 'stuttering personality' (your mental image of yourself) and its associated cognitive patterns and behaviours have been deeply ingrained over the years. Saying goodbye to this identity, no matter how uncomfortable or painful it has been, can feel daunting simply because it's so familiar and predictable. Our minds, after all, prioritize safety over everything else, and familiarity – even when it doesn't serve our happiness or growth – feels safe. Surprisingly, your mind's primary concern isn't your happiness or self-actualization but maintaining what it perceives as security. And yet, it's this very familiarity that can become the greatest obstacle to your growth.

Figuratively speaking, change can feel like a small death. But let me reassure you: it is not the end of you – far from it. In fact, it's a profound new beginning. As you journey further along the path of self-discovery, getting to know yourself more deeply, you'll come to see that the 'holding-back personality' you once believed was you – clung to and feared of letting go of – was never truly you. It was a rigid mental construct, much like a straitjacket. This construct was shaped by early experiences and later reinforced through the challenges and pressures of school, university, the workplace, relationships and life itself.

The process of dissolving stuttering should not evoke anxiety, as it's not about losing yourself. Rather, it's a journey of rediscovering your authentic self – of peeling away the layers that have kept you separated from your innate strengths and inner resources. These strengths, like hidden treasures, have long been buried beneath the rubble of fictitious narratives, illusions, false perceptions and imposed beliefs – ideas that were never truly your own.

Be gentle and patient with yourself as you move closer to your goal. Take time to notice and celebrate even the smallest shifts in your emotional states, reactions and behaviours. These incremental changes are not insignificant; they're meaningful milestones marking your progress on this transformative journey.

If someone else has found a way to overcome fear and anxiety – unlocking the joy, freedom and pleasure of genuine connection – then you can, too. Never doubt it. It's entirely possible, and you have every ability to join those who have already succeeded.

The reason so few people have conquered fear and anxiety is that only a small number have dared to imagine an alternative reality. These individuals have stepped beyond the boundaries of commonly accepted narratives. They refused to accept the rule that stuttering is incurable, choosing instead – whether through their own determination or the pressures of their circumstances – to disregard such scientific proclamations, no matter how persuasive or elaborate they seemed.

They've broken away from institutional limitations, taken full responsibility for their lives and begun forging their own paths. In doing so, they've achieved remarkable success. And so can you – provided you're ready to summon your courage and step beyond the comfort of familiarity.

Most PWS are deeply entrenched in institutionalized beliefs and perspectives. They place unwavering faith in certain scientific institutions to provide them with a solution, almost as if awaiting divine salvation that will one day descend upon them. They know the popular opinions on stuttering by heart, adhere to them almost religiously and often advocate for them with fervour. Yet, they seldom allow themselves to step outside these boundaries, to peek beyond the conventional narrative and explore alternative perspectives.

Their expectations are fixed on external solutions, relying on science to hold all the answers. In doing so, they remain trapped – though most don't even realize it. They assume that mainstream science alone is both the ultimate authority and the sole source of credible answers. What many fail to consider is that the answers often lie within us, waiting to be discovered. To access them, you must be willing to turn inward, to trust yourself and to grant yourself the permission to explore beyond the external. Authorize yourself to look within, and you'll find the truth!

Institutionalization creates a significant barrier to progress because it fosters uniformity, rigidly entrenched mental frameworks and, in some cases, ideologies. These frameworks, especially those resistant to change or evolution, act as mental traps, preventing growth and discovery.

This is precisely why so many fail to make meaningful progress towards freedom. Adhering strictly to the mainstream narrative about stuttering will not lead you to the destination you desire. You must muster the courage to step outside conventional ideas and break free from limiting beliefs. That is where the answers lie – and where your inner peace and freedom awaits.

Those who have made significant progress or eliminated stuttering altogether discovered the solution within themselves. But their journey began with a brave decision: they granted themselves the authority to question the norms and look beyond established opinions. You can do the same, and your journey to freedom can start today.

Here's a profound historical example of how simple, innovative ideas can face resistance when they challenge established norms – and yet, when applied, can lead to transformative solutions for seemingly insurmountable problems. The story of Ignaz Semmelweis, the father of hand hygiene, is a testament to the power of simplicity and a shift in perspective.

In the 1840s, Semmelweis observed a horrifying trend: women in maternity wards were dying of puerperal fever at alarming rates. Through careful observation, he discovered a troubling practice – doctors were moving directly from performing autopsies to delivering babies without washing their hands.

His solution was simple but ground-breaking: require handwashing with a chlorinated lime solution before any patient contact. Semmelweis didn't just address the symptoms, he pinpointed and tackled the root cause. The results were nothing short of miraculous – death rates plummeted from 18 per cent to just 2 per cent.

Despite the undeniable success, his idea was met with resistance. It challenged deeply ingrained practices and bruised the egos of many of his contemporaries. At the time, the germ theory of disease – which would later confirm his findings – was not yet understood or accepted. Semmelweis was ahead of his time, a pioneer who dared to challenge conventional wisdom for the sake of saving lives.

His story serves as a powerful reminder that small, humble changes, born of clear observation and a willingness to think differently, can alter the course of history. The answers we seek are often not found in complexity but in simplicity – waiting to be noticed, embraced and acted upon.

A simple solution, yet a profound effect. Ignaz Semmelweis's solution was as straightforward as it gets: 'Wash your hands!' Tragically, full recognition of this pioneering doctor's contribution came only after his death. Did they really need to wait that long? To sacrifice the lives of so many women before the medical authorities of the time could put their egos aside and accept his solution? It often starts with one person daring to challenge established beliefs. Semmelweis is just one example among many brave individuals across various fields who challenged the status quo and paved the way for progress.

I believe this story deeply resonates with and is directly applicable to debates about stuttering. It also introduced me to the concept of the 'Semmelweis Reflex', which describes humanity's tendency to reject new information that contradicts established beliefs. This reflex is another name for institutionalization – the very thing that affects many who stutter as well as the field of speech pathology, making the solution seem perpetually elusive.

The most impenetrable prison is that of the conditioned, egoic mind. It has no doors, no guards, no locks, no walls – yet you cannot escape it. As long as you refuse to look beyond your predicament and its surface-level symptoms, the solution will remain out of reach, appearing impossible. It's only when you begin to view the problem in a new and unconventional way that you finally see the door, open it and step into a reality where progress is indeed possible.

I hear you ask, 'If it were that simple, why don't people already know the answer and have the solution?'

Unfortunately, many people remain deeply unconscious, lulled into slumber by the demands of conventionality and the comfort of compliance. When you're unconscious, you're unaware. Looking beyond established beliefs requires not only courage but an extraordinary amount of determination. For some, the challenge is compounded by a fear of losing their sense of belonging to stuttering communities – a connection they hold dear.

Thankfully, I didn't face this dilemma. When I embarked on this journey, I wasn't part of any group. I had nothing to lose but everything to gain – and that's exactly what I did.

My hope is to empower you to help yourself: to truly understand how your predicament works, to observe it through the lens of your own daily life, and to learn how to navigate yourself out of turbulence and into balance – without the constant dependence on coaches, therapists or lifelong courses. In the worst-case scenario, if this approach doesn't work, you can always retreat to the familiar shell you've left behind. It will be there, waiting for you, if that's what you choose. But something tells me that if you've come this far – if you're reading this book – you won't want to go back. And most importantly, you won't need to.

The key to overcoming stuttering lies within you, as do all the treasures you seek.

The question is not 'why we stutter? But why we hold back'.

Why I Wrote This Book

The idea to write this book came to me spontaneously, inspired by the countless questions I have received about stuttering during individual sessions, online seminars and through various platforms over the past few years. These interactions shaped the main section of this book, which is written in a question-and-answer format. Each question approaches stuttering from a unique perspective, and the answers aim to provide comprehensive insights while encouraging deeper understanding and reflection.

Some answers are straightforward, while others are more reflective and may challenge deeply ingrained beliefs or traditional institutional notions about stuttering. If you find yourself feeling triggered or encountering mental resistance while reading, take it as a positive sign – it might indicate an opportunity for growth. Use this moment to pause and reflect, asking yourself: 'What belief am I holding on to? What am I resisting, and why?'

This book represents the heart of my holistic approach to addressing stuttering, as far as it can be captured in words. I want to express my deepest gratitude to the many individuals around the world who stutter and have brought their challenging questions to me. Their willingness to look beyond the surface, their curiosity and their commitment to self-discovery and inner transformation have been truly inspiring.

I am especially thankful for their courage to open their hearts, stay curious, listen with intention and apply what they've learned to their lives. Without their contributions, this book wouldn't exist. They're part of a small but steadily growing group of pioneers who are embracing alternative approaches to overcoming stuttering.

These remarkable individuals are reaching a deeper understanding of the anatomy of stuttering – its inner dynamics –and breaking free from the collective conditioned helplessness. They're moving beyond the widespread belief that stuttering is an incurable condition requiring complex solutions or centuries of research. Their journeys offer hope, and their courage lights the way for others to follow.

The answers are often closer than we imagine – right between your ears.

I trust that this book will find its way to those who are ready to embark on a profound journey of self-discovery and embrace this transformative approach. May it serve as a catalyst for their growth and healing. I also hope it reaches others, including speech pathologists, who may find its ideas thought-provoking and worthy of consideration. While they might not yet be prepared to fully embrace or practise these principles, perhaps the seeds planted through reading this book will, in time, begin to take root.

When that moment arrives, what once seemed complex and elusive may suddenly feel simple and self-evident. New possibilities and insights, long hidden in plain sight, will come into focus, revealing the path that was always within reach.

'You are stuck because of the way you look at the problem.'

— Olga Bednarski

What is Stuttering? The Alternative Paradigm

Stuttering is not merely a speech problem, as mainstream science often claims. At its heart, stuttering is an emotional challenge – one that goes far deeper than the mechanical act of producing words and sounds. In fact, the purely mechanical aspects of stuttering account for, at most, only about 5 per cent of the entire stuttering experience. Stuttering is a deeply ingrained habit, a learned response to emotional pain or trauma. Over time, this response becomes automatic – so embedded in one's identity that the individual is no longer consciously aware of how they are creating the stuttered speech.

In essence, people often become their stuttering. They believe they are 'it'. Over time, this experience shapes a mental image – a conceptual self – that evolves into what might be called a 'stuttering personality'. At its core, stuttering is also a spiritual challenge – a void that longs to be filled. The emotional problem, characterized by excessive control and resistance, acts as a barrier to filling that void. Its very existence stems from a disconnection from the self – a lack of inner awareness. As we explore this narrative together, you'll begin to see why this broader definition of stuttering is more accurate and how it intertwines with spiritual growth and self-awareness.

But let's begin at the root. Stuttering is a learned behaviour, an adaptation that originally developed as a response to the environment. It once served a purpose: shielding the individual from the potential harm of overwhelming emotional experiences within their social surroundings.

For a child, the emotional intensity of certain situations can feel unbearable. Most cases of stuttering begin in childhood, when a young mind simply can't process the raw, overwhelming emotions it's exposed to. To protect itself from emotional pain and potential psychological harm, the child unconsciously suppresses or represses these feelings. Over time, this suppression becomes a habit – a coping mechanism that, while adaptive in the moment, ultimately leads to a disconnection from the full expression of self.

What you're essentially suppressing is your true, authentic self – the part of you that was never fully validated, approved or accepted by the most important people in your life, such as your parents, caregivers, teachers and other authority figures. This validation was crucial for your survival. Unconsciously, you believed that by suppressing (or contracting, not allowing to expand, grow) or editing your true self, you could gain acceptance and love.

However, what happened as you tried to 'fit in' is that you became distorted. You moulded yourself into something other than your true essence, developing a persona and mindset that, over time, took root and now holds you back, no matter your age. This persona is not who you truly are, but rather an adaptation – an identity you created, even though it may feel real.

Ironically, it's often your thinking that keeps you trapped. Overthinking has helped shape a conceptual image of yourself – one that you've become deeply attached to. But in reality, this mental image only serves to separate you from your true self. If you continue to repress your authentic self, you'll remain disconnected from the very source of your unconditional happiness and personal power.

Another downside of emotional repression as a coping strategy is that it halts your emotional growth, leaving you emotionally frozen at the age when traumatic or adverse events occurred. At the time, whether in childhood or adolescence, you lacked the ability to process the emotional content of those situations. However, the emotional charge or trigger remains within you, often manifesting physically. Regardless of your current age, when you encounter certain situations or people, you may find yourself emotionally transported back to the past, reliving those emotions as if you're still that child. Emotional suppression stunts emotional growth, and I see this in many PWS: arguing, blaming, demanding, mistrusting and seeking external love and validation. Many are unwilling to take responsibility for their own healing and recovery.

Living in an adult world while emotionally remaining a child is confusing and unsettling. Life is for adults. When you truly mature emotionally, there comes a time when you no longer need external approval, validation or love because you can give that to yourself. You no longer feel the need to be perfect or 'good enough' in the eyes of others because you're no longer dependent on them for your sense of survival. When you grow emotionally, you become autonomous, in charge of your own life – and even the enjoyment of life becomes natural, as you stop attaching undue importance to events, especially those beyond your control.

Sometimes, external pressures ease or disappear – for example, when a child changes schools or an abusive parent leaves the family. In these cases, although there's no guarantee, the coping behaviour of emotional suppression (holding back) may no longer be necessary. It becomes redundant, and what were once minor verbal stumbles may naturally fade without the need for intervention or therapy. This is why some children are fortunate enough to outgrow the issue. Once stuttering becomes chronic and persists into adulthood, however, it transforms into something more than a developmental speech impediment.

Emotional conditions, such as speech anxiety, are highly dependent on specific situations and circumstances. This is why it's so difficult to pinpoint the exact cause.

At this point, you might ask: why doesn't stuttering develop in all children and adolescents who experience emotional trauma? Why does anxiety and emotional suppression manifest as stuttering or speech anxiety in some, but take a different form in others?

In many cases of stuttering, it's the child's personality that becomes scrutinized, judged or even physically punished by significant adults, leading to an assaulted sense of self. Typically, children who develop stuttering tend to be very active, expressive, loud and emotionally sensitive. They're easily overwhelmed by their emotions and wish to express them in an exuberant way – or in any way that may be deemed 'too much' or 'inadequate' by the standards of the adults around them. In response, parents may resort to emotional rejection, coldness, reprimands or even physical punishment.

A child who faces criticism, rejection and punishment from their parents – whom they see as their entire world – may unconsciously conclude, 'If my mum doesn't love me, I must not be good enough,' or 'I'm a bad boy/girl,' interpreting their parents' behaviour as a reflection of their own worth. This is because children see themselves through the eyes of their parents, and this perception can persist into adulthood, influencing not just those who stutter, but many people in various walks of life. Of course, this interpretation – a child's conclusion – is highly subjective and unconscious, based solely on the events they experience or witness. Due to their immaturity, lack of critical thinking and unawareness, children don't consider the wider context of family circumstances, financial struggles or relationship difficulties their parents may be facing. Instead, children are guided primarily by their emotional brains and judge experiences based on what they perceive 'as it is', taking events at face value.

When a child unconsciously concludes that they're 'not good enough' and internalizes this belief as their truth, they begin to reject and suppress parts of themselves in an attempt to avoid further punishment. They believe they're unworthy of love and approval, causing them to shrink and dim their own light. Ultimately, the primary instrument of expression for our personalities is our ability to speak.

When being yourself is believed to be punishable or unwelcome, the child experiences strong, often overwhelming negative emotions. In response, the child's natural instinct is to close up, suppress these emotions (choosing not to feel) and emotionally withdraw from the world in order to avoid causing displeasure and to steer clear of punishment or criticism. This emotional suppression leads to disconnection. Over time, speaking gradually becomes associated with anxiety, pain, fear, shame, discomfort, nervousness and even danger. In such cases, the wisest choice, from the child's perspective, is often to remain silent. What might have started as verbal hesitations or minor stumbles can, over time, evolve into full-blown blocks and obvious stuttering.

Parents (carers) who are not familiar with child development may mistakably assume that young children can't interpret their experiences or draw conclusions, thinking that children are 'living unconsciously', without the ability for rational or critical thought, and may even believe that they don't have emotions (these are not just anecdotal observations, but real points made by some parents). However, the absence of 'adult' logical (conditioned) thinking doesn't prevent children from making meaning or drawing conclusions about the world and the people around them – using their emotional minds instead.

As a child or adolescent encounters more difficulties, stuttering becomes a habitual, internalized behaviour – one that's memorized by the body and automatically recreated whenever the person finds themselves in a similar 'triggering' situation, setting or interaction with a particular person.

The influence of parents (carers) is critical

In young children, stuttering behaviour can be reinforced or intensified by anxious parents who place excessive emphasis on their child's speaking performance. Parents may become visibly upset or impatient when their child hesitates or mispronounces words, or they may take their child to various doctors in an attempt to 'fix' the issue. These actions can inadvertently signal to the child that something is inherently wrong with them – especially as they see their behaviour causing distress and anxiety for their parents.

In cases of late onset stuttering during adolescence, the situation becomes more complex. Beyond environmental factors and external pressures, self-reinforcement can exacerbate the problem. This includes overthinking, a negative self-perception, self-doubt, self-fulfilling prophecies, despondent inner dialogue and the tendency to imagine and mentally rehearse worst-case scenarios. These patterns, repeated over time, can solidify the experience of stuttering.

With repetition, what may have started as mere hesitations or minor stumbles becomes an ingrained learned behaviour, reinforced by the ongoing loop of negative inner dialogue. Once this behaviour is fully internalized, it becomes automatic, and the person loses conscious or rational awareness of how they're creating – and re-creating – the experience of stuttered speech.

As stuttering experiences accumulate across various social situations, the person's self-image – a conceptual mental image – becomes increasingly elaborate, distorted and convoluted. Layers of ideas, interpretations and conclusions are added on top of their lived experiences, giving shape to a persona or self-image that feels inseparable from who they are. Every positive and negative interaction further contributes to this mental map of reality, shaping a specific mindset.

In PWS, this mindset becomes what can be described as the 'mindset of stuttering'. This mindset is composed of deeply ingrained beliefs, ideas, inner narratives, attitudes, perceptions and reactions. Over time, it solidifies into a personality defined by stuttering, hypervigilance and disfluency – a role the individual comes to embody, often without realizing they have the power to step out of it.

The personality of stuttering – the role it plays in one's life – shapes a person's state of being. This emotional state persists daily, especially in speaking or social situations, but often extends beyond these moments, becoming an ongoing inner reality. It influences not only one's thoughts, feelings and emotional responses but also the way one interacts with the world. This inner climate – composed of recurring thoughts, emotions and reactions – ultimately moulds personal reality and life experiences, which some may describe as fate or karma. These patterns do more than maintain the mindset of stuttering; they also impact mood regulation, emotional well-being and even physical sensations in the body.

Feelings are powerful sources of information, deeply intertwined with the body. When you experience fear or anxiety, you don't just think, *'I'm scared.'* Your entire body responds (fills up), manifesting sensations that reflect your emotional state. You live the experience not only mentally but physically as well. For instance, fear translates into your body language and prompts you to slouch, tense your muscles, curl your toes, squeeze your buttocks, hold your breath or brace yourself as if preparing to fight, flee or freeze. Fear becomes an embodied experience – you become the fear.

Over time, the emotions tied to certain experiences – such as speaking in particular situations or interacting with specific people – are stored within the body, creating what's often called 'the memory of the body'. While you may not consciously recall the event or recognize the source of the tension, panic or muscular spasms, your body remembers. It re-creates or triggers the same response whenever you find yourself in a similar situation.

Over the years, this state of being and the mindset that drives it become second nature. You might be convinced that this is just who you are – that it's your temperament. I often hear people say they believe they're introverted, naturally shy, timid, unassertive or that they struggle with personal boundaries. But this isn't the case. These traits – shyness, perceived introversion, unassertiveness – are by-products of the specific personality you developed as an adaptation to your environment. Over time, this adaptation felt familiar and became your default.

The good news is that if this version of yourself no longer serves you, it can be changed. Imagine wearing clothes that once fit you as a child but now feel tight, restrictive and uncomfortable as an adult. You don't need to keep squeezing into them. You can choose a wardrobe that fits your current size, age, aspirations and preferences – one that allows you to move freely and comfortably.

What you've come to believe (and accept as truth) about your inherent personality is simply the result of all the adjustments you made to fit into your social environment. It only faintly resembles your true, authentic self – a watered-down version of the vibrant, expansive person you are at your core. Your full authenticity and potential are hidden beneath layers of false beliefs – `some handed down to you by others, and others you created yourself to make sense of why, for instance, you avoid social events or people. Yet, deep down, there might be a part of you yearning to connect, to participate and to feel part of a community.

You may believe that you had a perfectly happy childhood, but it's worth reflecting on the fact that none of us grows up in a highly conscious world. Even with the best intentions and efforts, no one escapes childhood without experiencing some level of emotional pain and suffering. Whether the challenges were extreme or more subtle, they left an impact. Strong emotional pain experienced during childhood or adolescence often follows us into adulthood, contributing to the development of a false persona – what we might call the '*stuttering personality*' – and the mindset that comes with it.

This mindset shapes our behaviours, influences our experiences and moulds our personal reality. Some aspects of this learned personality are so subtle and deeply ingrained that they escape the radar of conscious awareness. They operate quietly in the background, influencing our lives in ways we might not immediately notice or understand.

'You are not who you think you are! You are much more.'

— Olga Bednarski

The Circuit

Here is a brief overview of how it works: your thoughts (beliefs, views) shape your emotions, your emotions influence your bodily responses, reactions and behaviours, and your behaviours, in turn, shape your personal reality and the experiences you have. Speaking – whether it be fluently or disfluently, joyfully or hesitantly – is also an experience shaped by this cycle.

The journey of change begins by reversing this process, starting with a shift in your mindset – those habitual, repetitive thoughts. By changing your perspective and adopting a healthier, more compassionate view of yourself, others and the world, you can significantly improve your emotional regulation. This shift will positively influence your bodily reactions and behaviours, ultimately leading to entirely new personal experiences and a vastly improved quality of life – emotionally and in the way you express yourself through speaking.

I understand that the idea of change or letting go of something you've carried for a lifetime, can feel intimidating. You might even feel the urge to hold on tightly, fearing that letting go means losing yourself. But let me reassure you: the process of change is not about losing anything of true value. It's about releasing the layers of misconceptions, limitations and false beliefs that have clouded your life and held you back. It's about rediscovering and embracing your true self.

Change isn't about loss – it's about finding. It's not an ending, but a rebirth – a resurrection of your authenticity. It's a reconnection with the beautiful qualities and strengths within you that have been hidden, suppressed or forgotten. Change is about stepping out of the shadows and into the light!

No matter how you approach it, no matter how many theories or debates you explore, it all comes back to your mind. Your mind is the origin of all your experiences, including the experience of verbal self-expression – speaking.

'The mind is the source of all experience, and by changing the direction of the mind, we can change the quality of everything we experience.'

— Yongey Mingyur Rinpoche

The formation of our mindset begins within the family setting and continues to evolve as we move through life. Our minds are profoundly shaped by our environment, and the way we view ourselves and others is informed by the social panorama – the people who surround us. We often see ourselves through the eyes of those closest and most significant in our lives – our parents, caregivers, educators, friends and spouses.

Why is stuttering an emotional issue that reflects spiritual disconnection? It's because, as people learn to reject, deny, suppress or repress their emotions and disconnect from their feelings, they lose touch with themselves and their spiritual essence. This essence goes beyond the mind and beyond the conceptual self-image – it's the core of who we are, whether or not we consciously recognize or believe in it. This disconnection from our inner being often underlies many emotional, mental and relational challenges, including various addictions, depression and abusive relationships. Left unaddressed, this can deepen into what some describe as spiritual collapse.

Healing this disconnection involves reconnecting with oneself – not suppressing or rejecting emotions but embracing them. This means recovering your feelings and deepest emotions. When a person is ready to meet themselves with honesty and compassion, self-awareness begins to emerge, and healing (i.e. reconnection) follows. Self-awareness (via intentional observation) is one of the most vital steps in understanding and overcoming speech anxiety or any other life challenge.

As you observe, notice and begin to understand how you unconsciously create the experience of anxiety and blocking, you gain the power to change it. Awareness brings freedom. It offers you the opportunity to alter these patterns, reduce anxiety and eventually move past stuttering. This principle applies to almost any challenge in life: every problem carries within it the key to its own solution.

Once we become consciously aware of what's happening and why, the problem that may have troubled us for years can no longer control us. Control is returned to us, and we can choose to disengage from the problem and release it – if that's our desire.

No matter how you look at it, everything always comes back to the mind. Your thoughts (and mental images they evoke) hold incredible importance because they serve as the source of the information that shapes your personal reality. The quality of this information – whether benign or malevolent – determines the nature of your experiences. The conditioned mind is the root of all perception, and it's within the mind that the answers to our most pressing and heartfelt questions reside. Searching for external causes often leads to wasted time and frustration because all roads eventually lead back to oneself – to the mind and its content.

If you wish to change your experience – whether in speaking or any other area of life – you must start by changing the content of your mind. True transformation begins within. Until you change, nothing else can. This shift happens when you become more conscious and aware of your internal processes, the nature of your emotions and the patterns of your thoughts. Training your mind is akin to training a dog: with consistency and care, you can guide it to serve you well. The mind, when properly trained, becomes your servant and a powerful instrument – no longer your master.

As self-awareness grows, you'll begin to recognize the beliefs and ideas that no longer serve you – the ones that perpetuate fear and anxiety. By challenging, letting go of and replacing these outdated beliefs, you'll notice a profound shift. Your responses to situations and people will begin to change, not because the external environment has shifted, but because you have. This simple truth is common sense, yet it remains far from common practice. Many of us remain trapped by automatic, unconscious behaviours. It's time to make common sense a common practice.

As you identify and release limiting ideas and beliefs – those that cause blockages and stagnation in life, not just in speech – you'll notice transformations in your perceptions, reactions and behaviours. These changes ripple through all areas of your life, improving not only your verbal expression and social interactions but also your overall sense of well-being. You'll start to uncover and resolve the inner conflicts that have disrupted your life, undermined opportunities and led to self-sabotage.

For so long, you may have believed that these patterns were simply part of your personality, that they defined who you were. But, in truth, they were just the by-product of what you had come to believe about yourself (or what this world helped you to believe). Overcoming emotional challenges like stuttering is not just about speaking fluently; it's about reclaiming your life. It leads to a richer, more fulfilling existence through reconciliation – with yourself, with others, with your past and with the world at large.

'The motivation to overcome stuttering is not about satisfying the ego or forcing yourself to become someone you are not. Instead, it's about shedding everything that separates you from your true self and returning home. It's about reclaiming your authentic self along with the strongest personal qualities you've been suppressing all these years.'

— Olga Bednarski

How to Recover from Speech Anxiety: The Process

Since stuttering is a learned behaviour – a habitual coping response acquired through repetition, much like learning any other skill – it can also be unlearned. This unlearning happens gradually by adopting new beliefs and integrating them into your daily experiences. Over time, these new beliefs reshape your internal map of reality through consistent practice and repetition. This is why there's no 'magic pill' or quick-fix solution to dissolve stuttering – just as there's no 'fitness pill' to instantly give you a sculpted, muscular physique. Deep, lasting structural and behavioural changes require time, patience and dedication to fully assimilate and become part of your lived experience.

While great ideas and theories can be understood intellectually, intellectual understanding alone is not enough. Knowing something in your mind doesn't automatically lead to healing or liberation. For true transformation, knowledge must evolve into wisdom, and wisdom is born through lived experience. This shift occurs when you take what you've learned and apply it in real-life situations, allowing practice and exposure to new experiences to solidify your growth.

For knowledge to be effective, it must align with real-life experiences. Merely collecting and storing new information while continuing to act according to old patterns will hinder progress. Without practice, change remains a lifeless theoretical concept, far from being felt or realized in daily life. True growth requires moving beyond knowing something intellectually and actively engaging in the process to experience and embody the change.

Take learning to drive a car as an example. You don't become a skilled driver by merely reading about driving. Real understanding comes when you sit behind the wheel, practise and feel what it's like to navigate the road. In the same way, overcoming stuttering and achieving natural fluency requires applying what you've learned in real-life situations. Through practice and persistence, you'll unlock genuine growth and discover the freedom that comes with lasting change.

Having new experiences is an essential part of the journey towards dissolving stuttering. These fresh encounters gradually challenge and replace the old beliefs and perceptions you've carried and relied on for so many years. As you step into new situations, you don't merely think about change – you begin to feel it. Your experiences become more fluid and authentic, your fear of taking emotional (social) risks fades and your resistance gently melts away. You start to feel safer in your own skin, allowing your true self to shine through. This leads to greater openness, presence and natural fluency.

These new experiences reshape your internal map of reality, rewiring your brain so that speaking is no longer linked to fear, threat, shame or anxiety. Instead, speaking becomes something joyful, even something to eagerly anticipate.

This is how you evolve from the 'stuttering personality' – an identity rooted in holding back – to a 'personality of fluency', one that thrives in self-expression. With each new experience, paired with a positive emotional state, your body begins to internalize and embody this fresh emotional information. Over time, it learns to respond in a completely different way – one that's naturally aligned with fluency, confidence and the joy of self-expression.

Here are some illustrative examples:

- If you previously became physically tense and emotionally on edge, bracing yourself as if for impact before social encounters, you may now find it easier to consciously recognize and release that tension. Trusting yourself and relaxing into these experiences becomes more natural, allowing you to feel comfortable and at ease in your own skin.
- If you once slouched and avoided eye contact, you may now find yourself adopting a more open and confident posture, willingly meeting others' gaze.
- If your heart used to race and your palms grew clammy before speaking, you may now notice a growing sense of emotional control and calm presence.

Speaking becomes a safe and pleasant activity – not just in your conscious mind, but also within your body's memory. Fluency and confidence are achieved by moving past disfluency, releasing the habit of holding back and embracing peace, self-acceptance and authentic, fluid self-expression.

When searching the internet for solutions to stuttering, it often feels like navigating the Wild West. The landscape is flooded with countless products and companies offering so-called cures: snake oil remedies, herbal teas, ear devices and apps promising to end stuttering.

These products often rely on flashy marketing tricks, aiming to convince you of miraculous fixes. Whether it's a 'fast cure' or a device claiming to 'speak for you', these promises are often superficial and misleading. Other approaches suggest techniques to control or conceal stuttering, making social interactions less intimidating. While these methods may temporarily ease symptoms like blocking, they fail to address the deeper, underlying issue – the psychology of stuttering.

Neither quick fixes nor symptom-focused techniques resolve the core issue: speech anxiety rooted in the conditioned mind. The true key lies in working with the mind – challenging limiting beliefs, understanding one's psyche and learning to self-regulate emotional responses while recalibrating emotional states. This is the most natural, accessible and effective approach to overcoming stuttering.

Unfortunately, this method is overlooked by many PWS, including speech pathology, due in part to institutionalization. Institutionalization fosters sameness – a tendency to adhere to uniform approaches and ideas that may feel safe but rarely lead to breakthroughs. True success lies beyond conformity. It requires stepping outside institutional ideologies and principles, daring to embrace individuality and exploring novel paths that truly make a difference.

It's far simpler – and more fulfilling – to become acquainted with yourself, to introspect deeply and to learn how to regulate your emotions and thought patterns. This journey ultimately leads to mastery over your own mind. Mastery of your thoughts and emotions is one of life's greatest achievements. In contrast, placing empty hopes on some external force or an institution to 'magically cure' you overnight, or expecting the world to change and adapt to you, is unrealistic and disempowering. Many people cling to such hopes to avoid taking responsibility for their own lives, yet this mindset often results in frustration, despair and a sense of hopelessness.

Once you discover how to redirect your mind and take control of your inner world, the allure of snake oil remedies, magic pills or endless courses will fade. These so-called solutions will lose their appeal because you'll have gained something far greater and more valuable: the ability to regulate yourself and find stability during moments of turbulence or uncertainty.

It all begins with a willingness to look beyond stuttering and choose an alternative path – a path that has been successfully followed by those 'lucky few' who have managed to stop stuttering. The truth is, it's not about luck; it's about applying common sense and taking intentional steps forward. As the saying goes, 'Common sense is not yet common practice.' This book is here to help bridge that gap and guide you towards a life of greater confidence, ease, composure and self-expression.

'It's not that there isn't a solution. The solution is available right here and now. However, most people won't approach it, let alone use it, because it requires dissolving the ego and revealing their true essence – the perpetrator hidden beyond the veil of the problem. The ego cannot allow its own death.'

— Olga Bednarski

Why Do PWS Fail, and How Can They Succeed?

I've heard countless stories of failure, while success stories seem rare and far between. Yet, they do exist. With the rise of alternative therapies and the growing self-awareness among PWS, the number of successes appears to be steadily increasing. I consider myself one of those success stories. Unlike many others, I didn't endure an endless cycle of failed attempts or the despair that often accompanies them. From the very beginning, I made a firm resolution to succeed. Once I committed to the path of freedom, there was no turning back. Regaining my ability to express myself fully and eliminating anxiety were non-negotiable goals for me.

After spending 14 years immersed in the stuttering world and meeting countless individuals who struggled and failed, I couldn't help but ask myself: Why do so many fall short? What sets apart the few who succeed, myself included? Was it simply luck? Could it be that the causes of our stuttering were somehow different – perhaps easier to resolve – than most cases? Or does success depend on intellectual capacity or a unique ability to understand and process the problem?

Reflecting deeply, I've realized that those who succeed come from all walks of life and varied educational backgrounds. I've met academics and researchers of the highest calibre – brilliant minds with impressive credentials – and also successful, wealthy businesspeople who built thriving corporations. Yet, some of these individuals struggled to grasp the fundamental essence of their speech anxiety. On the other hand, I've encountered blue-collar workers, shop assistants and carpenters who, after just a few consultations, made remarkable progress.

These individuals showed a noticeable shift – not just in their speech but in their understanding of themselves, the mechanics of stuttering and the steps required to dismantle it. They 'got it'.

I can even point to at least three remarkable cases where individuals experienced significant improvement simply by absorbing the information shared in my videos. As one of them described it: '*I watched all of your videos, and one morning I woke up, and my stuttering was gone. At first, I thought my mind was playing tricks on me, but no – my anxiety and stuttering had actually disappeared!*'

Stories like this challenge the notion that overcoming stuttering requires one to be a maverick or a wunderkind. Extraordinary intellectual ability or status has little to do with achieving fluency. Success is within reach for anyone willing to engage with the process and apply what they learn with openness and determination.

So, what sets us – those who have overcome stuttering – apart? Were we simply more hardworking or dedicated than others? Did we desire freedom more intensely? Were we just better prepared or more ready to embrace change?

These questions have intrigued me because I do not consider overcoming stuttering to be inherently difficult – especially when the path forward is illuminated and the tools are readily available. With accessible psychological strategies, expert guidance from those who have walked this path, a clear sense of direction and answers to the key questions about stuttering, success feels entirely achievable.

So why, despite attending various courses or speech pathology programmes, do so many people still struggle? Why do they lose motivation, fail to make meaningful progress and remain bound by anxiety? What truly separates success from failure?

Stuttering becomes surprisingly straightforward to address and dissolve once you gain the right perspective. Unfortunately, acquiring that perspective is not always easy. The lived experience of stuttering often traps individuals in a mental and emotional box, restricting their ability to see beyond conditioned thoughts and feelings. This limited viewpoint can make freedom seem unattainable.

In writing this, I understand that I may challenge certain theories and scientific norms. However, I feel compelled to offer a perspective that breaks free of conventional constraints – a perspective that unboxes the brain and considers the emotional, physical and even spiritual dimensions of stuttering.

Driven by a desire to uncover the secret of success, I've spent the past two years actively observing and engaging in conversations across various platforms for PWS. Through these discussions and my personal journey, I've identified what I believe are the main reasons behind the inevitable failures many PWS encounter.

Reason 1: Focus solely on stuttering and speech

One of the most common missteps PWS make is directing all their attention to their speech – the external, visible symptom – while neglecting the deeper root causes of their speech anxiety, which lie within. These roots are intricately tied to their relationship with themselves, others, the world and their personal history.

Because speech is the outward manifestation of the problem, it's easy to become fixated on the blocks, repetitions and hesitations, all while ignoring the critical internal processes driving these symptoms. Yet, it's precisely these hidden inner dynamics – often overlooked or misunderstood – that trigger, sustain and reinforce the challenge. This lack of understanding leads many, even some of the brightest minds, to embrace the misguided belief that stuttering is an exotic, incurable disorder.

Let me be clear: if you stutter or experience overwhelming fear and anxiety in speaking or social situations, it doesn't mean you're 'sick' or broken. It simply reflects that your current relationship with yourself, others and the world might be misaligned or strained. And here's the empowering truth: this misalignment is not permanent. You have the ability to shift and transform it.

The quality of every relationship you have – whether with yourself, other people or the world – is determined by your thoughts and attitudes. At its core, this means your beliefs, ideas, narratives and ideologies actively shape how you perceive and respond to life. Dysfunctional or limiting beliefs inevitably result in strained or unhealthy relationships: with yourself, this might manifest as self-doubt, criticism or avoidance; with others, it might show up as anxiety, distrust or isolation.

Beliefs, whether empowering or limiting, functional or dysfunctional, are inherently self-reinforcing. Over time, they influence your reality, creating a feedback loop that seems to confirm their validity. For example, if you hold limiting beliefs such as 'life is hard', 'people are judgmental' or 'the world is unsafe', your experiences will align with these expectations, further solidifying what you already believe to be true.

To break free from anxiety and the stuttering it triggers and amplifies, you must first cultivate a healthier, more compassionate relationship with yourself. This is the foundation for true change. Without shifting the unhelpful attitudes you hold within, meaningful progress becomes impossible.

Many PWS struggle with a profound lack of self-love, often misunderstanding what self-love truly means. It's not vanity or selfishness, as some might believe. While this book can't explore the depths of self-love fully, the pages ahead will provide practical steps to dissolve any lingering self-loathing – whether conscious or not – and guide you towards genuine self-acceptance and inner peace.

As your relationship with yourself heals and strengthens, you'll notice that your connections with others and the world around you also begin to transform. This is because the distance we perceive between ourselves and others often reflects the distance we feel from ourselves.

Stuttering isn't merely a speech issue; it's a complex, emotional challenge rooted in the conditioned patterns of your inner world – your beliefs, perceptions and narratives, ideas about yourself, people and the world. To liberate yourself from stuttering's psychological grip, you must look inward, identify the thoughts and habits that no longer serve you and replace them with healthier, more empowering alternatives.

Focusing solely on speech – for example, trying not to stutter or attempting to control every word – ironically intensifies the problem. This approach often backfires because the more energy we devote to avoiding something, the more we magnify its presence in our lives. By fixating on the issue, we inadvertently invite the very outcomes we're striving to avoid.

One reason many people continue to struggle with stuttering is their reluctance to challenge conventional narratives. Those who have successfully overcome stuttering are the ones who dared to look beyond traditional explanations. They questioned the widespread belief that stuttering is an incurable 'condition' and stepped away from the idea that it must define them. When conventional therapies offered limited results, they sought alternative paths – and found success.

Belief plays a pivotal role in this process. Not belief in the religious sense, but as the expectations – whether positive or negative – that shape your path forward. Your beliefs and expectations influence your outcomes profoundly. Those who recover are the ones who refuse to be bound by the rules and limitations imposed by conditioned thinking. By rewriting their beliefs, they rewrote their reality.

To truly overcome speech anxiety, you must go beyond its visible symptoms and explore the deeper emotional landscape that fuels it. Stuttering isn't just about speech – it's about understanding and healing the inner workings of your mind and heart, addressing the fear and anxiety at its core.

The paradox is this: the path to fluency doesn't lie in obsessing over your speech but in transforming your relationship with yourself. And that's the wonderful truth!

Reason 2: Targeting the wrong goal: overlooking anxiety

This point underscores the importance of understanding the core issue. Focusing solely on speech – fixating on surface-level symptoms like blocking, repetitions or stalling – will not bring about the meaningful and lasting change you desire. You can't resolve a problem by addressing only its symptoms; you must identify and work on its root cause. Concentrating on speech alone is like masking pain with an anaesthetic while ignoring the underlying condition that causes the discomfort.

True progress begins when you address the root cause. It's then that those transformative improvements not only in speech but also in other areas of life – such as relationships, career and overall well-being – become possible. Stuttering, more accurately described as speech anxiety, is fuelled by underlying anxiety. The intensity of this anxiety varies from person to person and often corresponds to the severity of their stuttering.

This anxiety (which may manifest as mood swings, anger outbursts, acute perfectionism or excessively high expectations) often arises in everyday, non-threatening situations. Its origin lies within a person's internal 'map of reality'. This map is the mental framework through which we perceive ourselves, others and the world. It shapes how we interpret and respond to social environments. Tragically, this map often contains irrational beliefs and harmful narratives picked up during childhood – absorbed from influential adults or shaped by past emotional experiences.

Even if these formative events occurred years or decades ago, the emotional memories they created linger. As adults, when we face situations that remind us of those past experiences, the unresolved emotions resurface. We may find ourselves feeling just as vulnerable, frightened or overwhelmed as we did as children, even when the present moment poses no real danger.

Addressing the underlying anxiety is a vital step for every person who stutters. This journey involves:

- **Understanding yourself:** Take time to explore your thoughts, views, beliefs and emotional patterns.
- **Identifying harmful beliefs and ideas:** Notice the expectations, fears and assumptions that fuel anxiety, shame, guilt or unease.
- **Becoming conscious of your inner dialogue:** Listen to what you habitually tell yourself before, during and after speaking situations. This is especially important when things don't go as planned. Instead of harshly criticizing yourself for a perceived 'failure', nurture yourself with kindness, understanding and compassion.

When you address anxiety, detoxify and simplify your inner world, and learn to master your mind, you create a space of emotional safety and trust within yourself. This sense of inner security allows you to open up to the world with ease. As you find balance and calm within, your anxiety will naturally diminish, paving the way for a more confident and fluid self-expression.

Let me emphasize this once more: overcoming stuttering isn't solely about improving speech. It's about releasing everything that no longer serves you and embracing a more authentic, open and accepting version of yourself.

Reason 3: Lack of self-awareness: understanding your psyche, emotional triggers and tools for self-regulation

A lack of self-awareness – knowing how your mind operates, recognizing emotional triggers for anxiety and understanding the self-regulation tools that can help – often traps people in a cycle of frustration and despair. Many find themselves moving from one unsuccessful therapy to another, unable to break free because they lack insight into their inner world.

Lost in the coils of unconscious behaviour

Until you bring your behaviour into the light of consciousness (awareness), it will control you. But once you become aware of what triggers you, you can begin to self-regulate, dismantle and ultimately transcend the problem. This transformation goes beyond just improving speech – it reshapes your sense of self. It is akin to uncovering hidden layers of your being through a process of 'inner archaeology'.

Self-awareness is the cornerstone of meaningful change. Ignorance – a lack of understanding (unawareness) about what is truly happening within you – keeps old patterns firmly in place. When you focus exclusively on a single facet of yourself, like your speech, you miss the broader picture and the opportunity to understand yourself more deeply.

Most PWS struggle initially with self-awareness. They don't yet see how they unconsciously create and perpetuate their anxiety and stuttered speech. Their self-identity becomes confined to external markers – such as their name, age, gender, personal history, nationality, residence or, in the case of PWS, their way of speaking. This limited perspective often leaves them navigating life as if through a fog, disconnected from their deeper, truer selves.

The cycle of repeated mistakes

Without awareness, the same errors are repeated again and again. People grasp at 'just anything' in the hopes of improvement, often complicating their situation further and arriving at the same disappointing results. This unending cycle can lead to feelings of despair, hopelessness, anger and, tragically, even thoughts of giving up entirely.

Misunderstanding stuttering

Many people come to view stuttering as an enigmatic 'monster' that strikes without warning – an external force completely beyond their control. This perception blinds them to their own role in creating the internal sequence of events that culminates in stuttered speech. By misunderstanding the true nature of stuttering, they make the problem seem more daunting and unmanageable than it is.

The truth is this: the real barrier to overcoming stuttering lies in the absence of self-awareness – the inability to see how one's own mind generates the experience of holding back (or resistance). Once you begin to understand this connection, the path forward becomes much clearer and more attainable.

Waking up: a journey of self-discovery

For those of us who have overcome stuttering, the journey began with a profound awakening – breaking free from the illusion that we needed to 'fix' our speech. We rejected the societal narrative that stuttering is some mysterious, unchangeable genetic condition. Instead, we turned inward, focusing on understanding ourselves deeply. This meant diving into the inner workings of our minds to uncover the exact triggers and patterns that fuelled our anxiety and verbal struggles.

We came to realize that stuttering isn't merely a speech issue. It's a complex psychological process, deeply intertwined with our inner worlds. Addressing it required introspection, self-discovery and a willingness to face truths about ourselves. By carefully observing how our thoughts and emotions operated, we began to dismantle the false beliefs and limiting narratives that had held us captive for so long.

Through this process, we uncovered a vital truth: the experience of stuttering (as a behaviour) was something we had learned over time. It had become an ingrained part of our personalities. But here's the empowering revelation – what's learned can be unlearned. With awareness and intention, we could rewrite our narratives and choose a new way forward.

Mastery and transformation

By committing to mastering our minds and practising emotional self-regulation every day, we didn't just improve our speech – we transformed our entire lives. This newfound self-awareness rippled outward, enhancing relationships, careers and overall well-being. It wasn't just about communicating more freely; it was about letting go of inner resistance and living more fully.

Overcoming stuttering is, at its core, about understanding, regulating and ultimately liberating yourself. It's about embracing self-awareness as a powerful tool for creating lasting change and reclaiming the joy of authentic expression.

When you truly understand yourself and the nature of your challenges, you'll no longer take impulsive or desperate actions born from frustration. Instead, you'll approach your journey with clarity and purpose. You'll leave behind aimless detours and distractions, choosing instead to walk a deliberate and informed path towards the freedom and confidence you deserve.

Reason 4: What if there's a magic pill?

The belief in a 'magic pill' reflects immaturity – a reluctance to take full ownership of one's life and a desire to place responsibility in the hands of an external saviour. This mindset can leave you vulnerable to exploitation by those who offer grand promises, claiming they can 'cure' you in a matter of days. To truly progress, this hope for a quick, miraculous fix must be let go, replaced with a mature and resolute commitment to taking charge of your recovery.

The persistent dream of a 'one-day magic pill' is one of the most significant barriers preventing many from overcoming stuttering. It keeps people in a holding pattern – waiting, hoping and deferring action. As a result, they postpone their lives, careers, relationships, joy and happiness indefinitely.

The sooner you realize that your recovery – and your life – rests in your own hands and begin taking deliberate, meaningful steps towards the life and speech you desire, the sooner you'll experience the transformation you seek. Along the way, you'll uncover valuable insights about yourself, others and the world. The journey isn't just about the destination but also about the incredible growth and self-discovery you'll experience. It's a process to be embraced, not rushed. Overcoming stuttering (or anxiety) is a personal journey, and while there are no shortcuts, this should not be disheartening. Instead, it's a reason to rejoice – because the path itself is rich with lessons and rewards.

An extraordinary case: Paul Stamets and the magic of mushrooms

Paul Stamets' remarkable experience with psilocybin mushrooms offers an exceptional example of reverse learning – unlearning stuttering or 'holding back' through a single transformative event. His story illustrates how stuttering, a conditioned response developed and reinforced through repetition, can sometimes be undone in extraordinary circumstances.

According to Paul's account, after consuming 20 grams of psilocybin mushrooms while walking in the woods, he climbed to the top of an oak tree. Shortly after, a lightning storm erupted, creating an emotionally and neurologically intense experience. This dramatic event seemed to 'reset' his neurological pathways, resulting in an immediate cessation of stuttering and the absence of fear.

This instant transformation occurred without the need for repetition or practice because of the overwhelming emotional intensity of the experience. The combination of the psychedelic journey, the danger of the storm and the spiritual significance of the moment created a powerful catalyst for change. Paul described the event as both deeply spiritual and terrifying – he feared for his life as lightning flashed around him, shaking him to his very core.

Such emotionally charged experiences have a unique power to rewire the brain and eliminate entrenched habits or behaviours. Similar phenomena can sometimes be observed in other areas, such as smoking cessation following a life-threatening health scare like a stroke. These events can trigger immediate and profound behavioural shifts by disrupting old patterns and establishing new, healthier responses.

This is what happened to Paul. I delve deeper into the concept of reverse learning in my first book, *The Anatomy of Stuttering* (Bednarski 2022). However, it's important to understand that Paul's experience cannot be replicated – the circumstances unfolded naturally, in a way that defies duplication. So, please, don't try this at home.

Reason 5: Secondary gains of stuttering

I know this may sound surprising or even nonsensical to many PWS, but over time I've noticed that there are secondary gains associated with stuttering. These gains can cause even those who truly want to overcome stuttering to unconsciously hold on to it, sometimes even defending it when a workable solution or an ex-stutterer offers a way out.

The most prominent secondary gains, which are often interrelated, include the following:

First, stuttering can sometimes be perceived as a valuable personality trait – '*a cute little thing*' that defines who I am and makes me more appreciated or worthy of attention, often from those who nurture or care for me.

The second gain stems from the fear of losing a sense of belonging (attachment). For some, stuttering may tie them to a group of like-minded individuals, such as others who also stutter. If they improve their speech and move away from this group, they might fear rejection from those who remain in the stuttering community. Friends who continue to stutter may feel threatened by this change, sometimes opposing the idea of 'recovery' out of fear or jealousy. PWS often express a fear of losing emotional closeness with relatives or friends if they change how they speak or present themselves.

The third gain comes from holding on to the belief that stuttering is a genetically inherited disorder. This belief reinforces a victim mentality, shifting the responsibility for recovery away from the individual and placing it on external factors, like an intolerant society or overbearing parents. When someone sees speech anxiety as an incurable, genetic condition, they may adopt a martyr-like perspective. This belief brings with it a sense of heroism and perceived 'specialness' for living with the condition, which, as odd as it may seem, can offer a strange sense of satisfaction. It can create an emotional connection to the struggle, almost like a bittersweet comfort, making it harder to break free.

We unconsciously hold on to these so-called secondary gains because, strangely, the restrictions in our lives – whether they're stuttering, unsatisfactory relationships or loneliness, etc. – offer a sense of safety and predictability. Even though we may consciously desire change, the thought of it can feel unsettling. Humans bizarrely derive pleasure from their suffering. Change opens the door to the vast unknown, and the uncertainty it brings can be intimidating and therefore uncomfortable, leaving us to question what lies beyond the comfort of the familiar, even if that familiar place is unsatisfying.

Here's an illustrative example: imagine you've always been socially avoidant and didn't have many friends. People generally showed little or no interest in you. Then suddenly, everything changes – people start showing genuine interest, approaching you, wanting to connect and get to know you better. Honestly, after years of introversion and social isolation, how would this change make you feel? I'm sure you would feel nervous, maybe even overwhelmed. Change, no matter how positive, can be uncomfortable at first. But remember – discomfort is temporary. As the new reality settles in, it gradually becomes your natural norm.

The key is not to resist. Do not dig your heels in or fight against the change, as doing so only creates unnecessary delays and added suffering. Instead, resolve to trust and allow the change to unfold naturally. Take a deep breath, embrace it with gratitude and trust that life is guiding you in the right direction.

All of the secondary gains I've described point to an adaptation – a coping mechanism or defence against losing something that feels unique, valuable, safe and even central to one's identity: '*Who will I become without my anxiety and stuttering?*' Stuttering, in this case, helps individuals feel accepted, loved and recognized within their community.

Who would want to let go of something that made them feel special, safe, unique or even heroic? Something that fostered relationships and provided a deep sense of belonging to a 'special' group? Naturally, no one would. This is why stuttering, as a conditioned trait, is often fiercely defended and protected. The mere thought of releasing it – of recovering – no matter how rationally understood, can stir intense anxiety and unease. The uncertainty about what lies on the other side of letting go feeds the urge to 'hold back', keeping one from taking meaningful steps forward, even when those steps could lead to profound improvement. The perceived benefits of staying the same often lead to the rejection of help or advice, even when it's offered with care and without conditions. Clinging to the familiar feels safer than stepping into the unknown.

As I've mentioned before – and will continue to emphasize throughout this book – what awaits beyond letting go is not a loss of any kind (except perhaps the loss of illusions), but a profound and genuine gain: the reconnection with your true, authentic self and expansion that is '*unpacking*' of your, up until now, unexpressed potential. It's about clearing away the mental clutter that has made your life feel small, fearful, constrained and uneventful. In doing so, you'll unlock access to the extraordinary inner powers and resources that have always been within you – dormant, hidden, but never lost. Through this process, you'll discover not just who you are but also who you are not. Many PWS, like so many of us, sit atop vast mines of unexpressed personal potential – gold and diamonds – but never enjoy these riches because they remain buried beneath layers of '*informational and conceptual clutter.*'

Then, there's the idea of 'stuttering pride', which can feel deeply appealing to some. In essence, it's just another conceptual identity. Although it 'legitimises' stuttering and has a positive twist, it can be just as limiting.

It offers not only a sense of belonging to a 'special' group or tribe (a source of connection and attachment) but also the much-desired experiences of attention, validation and even admiration – particularly within communities of PWS. To be validated and unconditionally accepted is a profoundly healing experience. For many PWS, especially those who may otherwise feel socially isolated or lonely, this acceptance can serve as a cornerstone of emotional well-being. It becomes a vital source of comfort and meaning in life, and for some it can feel essential to their very survival.

Richard Parent, a respected figure in the stuttering community and a speech coach, shares his perspective on the matter: '*Those who advocate such ideas forget that stuttering represents only one percent of the population. They also forget that, for most PWS, stuttering is real suffering. That being said, I acknowledge that some cases of stuttering are particularly severe. In such situations, it is crucial for society to provide accommodations, ensuring that even those with the most challenging forms of stuttering can contribute meaningfully and earn a living, rather than being relegated to a life dependent on social welfare. There is nothing more disheartening than that.*'

What's concerning is how this campaign, despite its well-meaning intentions, risks fostering a division that perpetuates an 'Us/Disfluent vs Them/Fluent' mindset. When politicized enough, it can quickly escalate into an ideological conflict – 'us against them'. As you might imagine, this dynamic doesn't build bridges of understanding; instead, it creates fertile ground for misunderstanding, distrust, resentment and even further social fragmentation.

Occasionally, I come across enthusiastic (or flaunting) remarks in online stuttering communities, such as, '*I stuttered and blocked during the meeting, and I loved it.*' While I wholeheartedly support acceptance, and it's truly beautiful to see someone embrace their stutter without making a big deal of it, these types of comments often raise a question. True acceptance doesn't typically seek attention, praise or approval in this way.

Individuals who have genuinely come to terms with their stutter don't place it at the centre stage of their lives. If anything, they downplay it and carry on. I've even observed cases of people with severe stutters who seem to have reconciled so completely with their unique trait that they scarcely think about it. At least, that's the impression I've got as an observer. They've embraced their stutter in a way that feels natural and unforced.

How can I tell when someone has truly accepted their stutter? It's when negative emotions no longer cling to it. They've moved on to a deeper, more profound level of acceptance. They don't hold back out of fear or demand validation from others. They transcended their predicament and simply live their lives as they are, authentically and freely. However, such individuals are the exception rather than the rule. And as the saying goes, exceptions prove the rule. For the vast majority of PWS – even those with relatively mild cases – their stutter is a source of significant anxiety, discomfort and a barrier to life opportunities, whether in relationships, careers or other areas of personal growth. Most of these individuals don't want to hear about acceptance – they want to overcome it.

Ideas such as 'stuttering is just another way of speaking' or 'stuttering with confidence' can feel like comforting ways to cope – a socially supported justification that offers psychological relief and support. While these approaches have their positive aspects, such as offering validation, they can sometimes act as a form of self-deception. They may inadvertently keep a person anchored within their '*inner world of anxiety*', preventing them from exploring their true potential and discovering the richness of life beyond their perceived limitations.

This mindset, while well-meaning, may close the door to many opportunities for a fulfilling and meaningful life – forming deeper relationships, pursuing a career that resonates with one's talents, finding inner peace and building genuine confidence to face life's challenges head-on. Instead of managing obstacles with resilience, this perspective may lead to avoidance and an over-reliance on comfort zones.

The '*packaged ideology*' of stuttering acceptance, while intended to soothe and empower, can sometimes cultivate learned helplessness or a sense of forced self-acceptance. It's a bit like indulging in fast food – it's quick and satisfying in the moment but, when used as a substitute for nourishing meals, can lead to unintended consequences such as poor health and extra pounds.

In this context, the word '*acceptance*' often becomes a superficial mental label – a way of rationalizing the situation rather than genuinely resolving it. It might create the illusion of peace on the surface but, beneath that, feelings of resistance and unhappiness linger. True acceptance requires more than saying, 'I'm okay with this.' It involves releasing the emotional and mental patterns that perpetuate control, frustration and discomfort. Without addressing these deeper layers, many who claim to have 'accepted stuttering' may still find themselves stuck in cycles of dissatisfaction and emotional struggle.

Genuine acceptance is undeniably challenging, especially when stuttering feels exhausting and drains a person's energy. The physical manifestations, like facial twitches or contortions, can add to this difficulty. Additionally, social misunderstandings and missed opportunities to connect with people beyond the PWS community can amplify feelings of isolation. It's important to recognize that stuttering, in and of itself, is neutral. The discomfort it causes stems from the disruption it creates and the meaning we attach to it.

As you already know, stuttering is a learned behaviour – essentially a coping strategy – driven by chronic emotional suppression. When emotions are suppressed (i.e. contracted), authenticity is also repressed, which stifles emotional growth (i.e. expansion or growth). Life is a game, but it's a game for adults, and to be an effective and fearless player one must mature emotionally. Clinging to the idea that 'stuttering is just another way of speaking' may offer a sense of psychological safety and predictability – 'let's keep things as they are' – and can feel like a perfectly rational justification within PWS communities. However, this ideology often hinders personal growth, emotional maturation and independence. In the long run, it deprives individuals of so much more. It keeps you stuck and blinds you to how expansive and fulfilling your life could truly be.

The sense of control that many PWS seek (and fear losing it) unfortunately doesn't come from maintaining the status quo or from external societal acceptance or validation. After all, you'll always encounter someone who doesn't understand or empathize. True control, contentment and peace of mind come from mastering your emotional life and inner world. This isn't merely forced control that stems from fear of losing; it's mastery.

Mastery is achieved by becoming deeply attuned to your authenticity and dis-identifying from the false, egoic personality – the personality shaped by stuttering or holding back. You become the skilled captain of your life's ship, able to steer and course-correct at will, even amidst turbulence. And yes, you will face turbulence. Mastery doesn't imply perfection, nor does it guarantee a challenge-free existence. Instead, it provides inner peace, genuine unconditional self-acceptance and the strength to support and appreciate yourself – even when others do not.

Mastery is a hallmark of adulthood (i.e. full emotional maturity, and/or rootedness in your being). Unlike children, who are often led and told what to do, adults cultivate their own sense of agency and self-governance.

As you'll see in the questions below, for the majority of PWS, 'acceptance' of stuttering or 'stuttering with confidence' is not a viable option. Speech anxiety causes significant emotional distress and disrupts careers, relationships, mental health and more. As long as stuttering continues to cause suffering, the idea of 'true acceptance' may sound appealing but will remain largely hollow and unattainable.

For those who doubt the existence of secondary gains, I want to share that I once denied them too. I wouldn't have believed in their presence had I not heard others describe them at length – hesitating or consciously choosing to leave things unchanged for the reasons mentioned above.

And that's okay. There's nothing inherently wrong with choosing not to change. But if you take this path, it's important to truly accept your 'unique trait' without blaming or resenting society for not always understanding, accommodating or celebrating it. Once you genuinely embrace your stuttering and let go of the need to make it the focal point of your life, you may find that the mental chatter surrounding it begins to fade. You'll no longer be interested in making it a 'big deal'.

'Whatever problem or ailment you might have is not independent of your personality. To overcome it, your personality must evolve into one that is free from the problem. It can be done!'

— Olga Bednarski

Reason 6: Blaming the genes

I have never been convinced by the idea that stuttering is purely genetic, no matter how much scientific evidence is presented to support it. This is because other studies clearly show that genetic expression is deeply influenced by the environment we live in. Our environment signals our genes, shaping how they manifest, and ultimately we become products of our surroundings. Stuttering, as I see it, is a learned coping mechanism that developed in response to the stressors we encountered. At some point in our lives, this self-repression – manifesting as stuttering – served a purpose. It felt safer to repress rather than express – whether that meant hiding true feelings, emotions, needs or authenticity.

For example, when I was in school, I concluded it was better to stay quiet than risk being ridiculed or humiliated in front of the entire class. This decision, born of self-preservation, only deepened the problem. My acute emotional sensitivity and hypervigilance to social dynamics heightened the dilemma and made speaking feel even riskier.

Interestingly, the moment I stepped out of the school gates, a brighter, more social version of myself would suddenly emerge. My body language, facial expressions, vocal tone – everything shifted. It was like stepping into a completely different role. Looking back now, I realize I was playing two distinct social roles: one for school (public) and one for after-school (private). It was as if I were switching costumes, depending on where I was. These roles were my adaptations – my defence strategies for navigating two very different environments.

The only 'stuttering gene' for most PWS seems to be the inherent sensitivity passed down from their parents – a predisposition to anxiety and heightened emotional awareness. I discuss this in detail in my first book, *The Anatomy of Stuttering*. This inherited sensitivity makes PWS hypervigilant to facial expressions and subtle social cues, far more so than people who are less sensitive.

As for brain scans often cited in research, it's important to note that chronic stress and emotional repression leave tangible, detectable marks on the brain. The stress a child or adolescent experiences while trying to fit in, be 'normal' or avoid disappointing significant adults can physically shape their brain. There's substantial research supporting this. Stress changes our bodies, especially when it's chronic. Emotional repression has profound implications for our physical and mental well-being.

Stuttering did not originate in the brain – it began as an adaptation to life experiences.

Another example often labelled as an incurable genetic condition is ADHD (attention deficit hyperactivity disorder), characterized by tuning out and restlessness. Once again, because physicians lack a comprehensive explanation for it, they frequently default to calling it incurable. But if we look closer, ADHD can also be understood as a coping mechanism. Why and when would someone tune out? Often, it's when they feel emotionally overwhelmed, unable to process or cope with their surroundings. In the case of stuttering, the defence mechanism manifests as holding back – self-suppression.

Mainstream medicine is undeniably powerful and has brought us countless benefits, but it also has significant blind spots. One of its greatest limitations lies in its poor acknowledgement of the profound connection between emotions and mental or physical health. This oversight can be maddening to contemplate. Fortunately, there are small but meaningful shifts happening. Some doctors are beginning to ask patients about their life stresses, recognizing the interplay between emotional and physical well-being. Still, the medical profession has traditionally operated on the belief that the body and mind are separate, independent entities – a view that's outdated and deeply flawed.

If research into stuttering is built on the premise that emotions play no role in its development, its conclusions are inherently limited. Remove the notion of pathology from stuttering for a moment, and instead consider yourself within the broader context of your life. Start from childhood and examine how you've learned to adapt to the challenges you faced. Stuttering, like many behaviours, didn't emerge in isolation; it evolved as part of your response to the world around you.

On another note, I've witnessed (in some, unfortunately, participated) many heated debates in online forums and support groups between those who reject the idea of stuttering as a neurological condition and those who uphold it. These exchanges make me wonder: why do individuals who firmly believe that stuttering is incurable invest so much energy in seeking methods or arguing their point? If they truly accept that stuttering is 'incurable', then their path forward seems clear – a lifetime of acceptance. So why waste time attempting to discredit those striving for solutions and personal growth? Could it be that, deep down, they harbour doubts they're unwilling to admit?

In many support groups, there seems to be an intentional effort to prevent members from asking deeper questions, exploring new ideas or stepping beyond what's immediately visible. Shielding people from information that could potentially help them alleviate their suffering feels, to me, like an act of harm. Some may justify this by claiming they're protecting individuals from the discomfort of failure or the pain of dashed hopes. But in doing so, they're also protecting them from truly living.

Yes, life can be uncomfortable and even painful when you grow, expand, evolve and push past your limitations. But discomfort and growth are essential parts of living. They do not destroy us – they shape us. Nobody should shield you or me from the beautiful, messy and sometimes challenging experience of life.

When people begin to question, the mental box – the constructed belief system – starts to crack and break apart. This is when the way out begins to reveal itself, offering the possibility of freedom. However, in most support groups, the structure often seems designed to keep people's attention fixed firmly on the problem. The discussions are intentionally steered towards reinforcing the issue, never allowing individuals to look beyond it. In this way, the problem is perpetuated and even strengthened.

It feels as though people's heads are being held underwater, and when they attempt to lift them, someone forcefully pushes them down again. To me, this is deeply concerning. Just imagine: a stranger, perhaps a group administrator, assumes the role of authority, deciding your fate by policing what you can read, explore, discuss and see. Who authorized these individuals to make decisions for you or me? Doesn't that worry you?

If I were to discover that someone was withholding information that could potentially help me, I would feel not only concerned but furious. This gatekeeping prevents growth and keeps people trapped in their suffering. Stuttering research, unfortunately, often searches for answers in the wrong places, remaining stuck in an outdated paradigm. Western medicine has historically separated the mind and body, failing to view stuttering – or many so-called 'incurable ailments' – as interconnected phenomena. While I've heard that this perspective is beginning to shift, the oversight is still significant and hampers progress in the field.

Dr Paul Brocklehurst, author of *The Perfect Stutter* and a respected voice in the stuttering community, shared his thoughts on stuttering research in our correspondence. He said, 'Most stuttering researchers and clinicians are simply unaware of what they don't know. There is very little financial reward in stuttering research. The NHS does not provide them with the support they need after they qualify; they do not even have access to proper academic journals and research.'

This is why I believe that scientific inquiry should not be reserved solely for institutions. If it is, it risks becoming dogmatic – another form of religion. Instead, each of us has the right to explore and investigate the phenomena that affect our lives. Good science begins with careful, honest observation, and that's something we're all capable of doing. I hope you agree that no one should take on a parental role, deciding for you what you can read, explore or follow. Mental health is deeply personal, and so is the path you choose to heal. It's disheartening to see that suffering often persists simply because people are not allowed to ask questions or seek alternative answers. I don't like to see unnecessary suffering. This is why I do this work.

Once you begin to question and inquire, you can no longer be easily misled. Clarity will start to emerge, freeing you from the grip of popular opinions and making you less susceptible to external control. Curiosity and inquiry are like rays of sunlight, dissipating the darkness of confusion. And the art of inquiry is available to every one of us, right here and now.

As you begin to ask questions, the fog of ignorance and doubt – those heavy clouds that may have loomed over you for years – will start to lift. Through the gaps, a clear blue sky will appear, followed by vivid, golden rays of sunlight. This light represents the truth and the healing knowledge that will illuminate your path, guiding you towards an alternative way. With this clarity, you'll begin to see the way out and find the freedom that has always been within your reach.

I deeply dislike witnessing suffering in the world, and I know that stuttering causes real pain. The purpose of my work is to help lift that burden, to show people that they too can take charge of their lives and move towards true healing and reconciliation.

'The motivation to overcome stuttering has nothing to do with ego or seeking perfection. It's an inner drive to free yourself from the psychological shackles that hold you back and return to your authentic self – free, light, joyous, resilient, and fulfilled.'

— Olga Bednarski

Reason 7: The romantic ideation of stuttering as a valuable karmic lesson

The idea that overcoming stuttering – or any form of restriction – is merely a desire of the ego, a sign of alleged 'unacceptance' and that wanting to change is somehow 'bad', suggests that stuttering is a karmic lesson one must endure to earn paradise in the afterlife. This notion couldn't be further from the truth. Stuttering, as a mind-made predicament, arises from an unhealthy ego. The desire to overcome it is not a superficial whim or lack of self-acceptance but a deep spiritual longing to return to a natural state of peace, bliss and joy – our inherent states of being, not suffering.

Ego is a sticky, tenacious thing, capable of convincing you of anything to maintain its control. It thrives on mental rationalizations, weaving elaborate stories to prevent you from becoming who you're truly meant to be. Overcoming stuttering isn't about struggling against yourself or striving to become someone you are not. Quite the opposite: speech anxiety separates you from your true self and veils your authentic essence. The journey to overcoming it is about shedding what you are not, stepping back into your authenticity and becoming more and more fully yourself.

I know many of you reading this have tried various methods and worked tirelessly to find success. But perhaps that's why you haven't yet succeeded. If something feels unbearably hard, it often means you're approaching it the wrong way. You may not yet fully understand the nature of your problem, or you may be overcomplicating it, turning it into a high mountain that feels impossible to climb.

When you step onto the right path and grasp the true essence of your challenge, progress becomes swift, even joyful – like playing a game. The obstacles you once saw looming before you will dissolve. Believe me, there are no physical barriers in your way. The only real obstacle is the conditioned mind (the ego), which stubbornly pulls you deeper into confusion, creating dramas and distractions to keep you stuck.

The (undisciplined) mind loves to create problems, revel in its own suffering and spiral into endless tears.

I've observed that those who have successfully overcome stuttering are often met with scepticism or even discomfort when they talk about the possibility of breaking free from it. This makes me wonder: are people truly ready to let go of the problem, or are they holding on to it?

For some, stuttering may have become so ingrained in their identity – the 'personality of stuttering' – that they can't imagine life without it. Perhaps they fear losing a part of themselves, as though letting go of stuttering would feel like losing an arm or a leg.

But let me say this clearly: there's no loss involved. On the contrary, overcoming stuttering offers a profound gain – a life filled with greater clarity, inner peace and a deep sense of reconciliation. As I often remind people, overcoming speech anxiety is about much more than just speech. Stuttering is a learned behaviour, a coping mechanism rooted in self-suppression. It separates you from your true self, and the desire to overcome it is a natural yearning to reconnect with who you are at your core.

This journey is not about striving to become someone else; it's about rediscovering and reclaiming the person you've always been beneath the layers of fear and mental conditioning. As you let go of what's not truly 'you', you naturally become more authentically yourself. It's a process of love, of peeling back the layers to reveal your essence.

In the end, it all comes down to personal choice: to remain in the familiar shadows or step into the light. Neither choice is inherently good or bad; they're simply paths, and you have the right to choose your own direction. Just remember, every choice carries its own consequences, shaping the life you create for yourself.

'Whatever you believe about yourself, you will consciously and unconsciously strive to prove to yourself.'

— Olga Bednarski

Reason 8: Wanting quick results, the 'fast-food culture' and one-and-done solution

There are no quick fixes or 'three-day cures' when it comes to overcoming stuttering. The process of acquiring stuttering took time, becoming ingrained through repeated patterns of thought and behaviour. It has been the somatic body experience. Similarly, unlearning stuttering requires time and patience. Stuttering is a learned behaviour, and unlearning it follows the same principle: repetition. The journey begins by adopting new beliefs, ideas, and perspectives, then gradually integrating them into your daily life until they become your new reality.

This aligns beautifully with the Hebbian rule in neurophysiology, which states, 'Nerve cells that fire together, wire together.' Repetitive thoughts, emotions and actions form a closed neural structure in the brain, directly shaping your everyday experiences. Whether your reality is one of stuttering or flowing speech, it's a reflection of the neural circuits you've built over time.

How does this apply to stuttering? If you consistently harbour negative thoughts about yourself – viewing yourself as inferior, fearing being 'found out' because of your speech, seeing others as critics, or anticipating failure in social situations – these thoughts form a neural circuit. This circuit triggers corresponding emotions and behaviours, creating a reality in which you indeed fail, block and feel ashamed or less than others. Over time, this cycle reinforces itself, making the problem feel inescapable.

But here's the good news: this cycle can be broken. You have the power to create a new reality. The first step is to 'awaken' – to become conscious and aware of the current patterns you're perpetuating and the consequences they bring. Awareness is the key to transformation. Once you're aware, you can begin creating a new reality of inner peace, flow and comfort. This begins by deliberately choosing to circulate life-affirming, positive thoughts in your mind.

With consistent repetition – at least three months of daily practice, such as listening to mindset audios and engaging with self-help tools (many of which you can find on my channel) – you can begin to reshape your neural pathways as well as somatic (i.e. bodily) reactions. These new patterns of thought and belief will gradually form a new closed neural structure, a kind of mental 'software' that supports new, empowering experiences of speaking.

An important point to remember is that the meditations (or mindset audios) you choose must deeply resonate with you. You need to truly feel them and embrace everything they convey as your truth. Only then can they create the desired effect. You must believe what you hear and make the ideas your own. This means living according to these new ideas. Positive affirmations alone, if they don't resonate with you, won't help – they remain on the surface level of rational understanding and never reach your subconscious mind.

If, despite listening to positive affirmations, you still find yourself feeling, mindlessly reacting and behaving in the same old ways, it's a sign that positive thinking alone isn't working for you. This is why I don't believe in simply repeating statements you don't believe in. You can't just say something you don't feel and expect transformation. The subconscious mind is best accessed through your emotions, so it's essential that you feel emotionally moved when selecting and engaging with your meditations.

Your self-help tools can also include books filled with ideas (ideologies) that resonate with you. It's important to revisit these books multiple times, allowing intervals between readings for information to take root. Each time you go back to them, you'll discover new insights – something you may have missed or not fully grasped the first time.

As you introduce new ideas and beliefs into your mind, your brain – and then your entire being – will begin to assert your new reality. This reality reflects the life you truly want to live. The more often you activate the same neural pathways by choosing to respond differently in various situations, the more your brain aligns with this new reality. Suddenly, you'll find yourself more open to meeting new people, embracing new experiences and feeling excitement rather than dread before a phone call or presentation. You'll begin to feel pleasant anticipation instead of panic.

Over time, your thoughts will expand beyond their old limitations. A greater number of neural connections will be activated, offering you more options for how to respond to life's events and challenges. From these new patterns, a refreshed mental profile emerges – a personality grounded in fluency, composure and improved mental well-being.

Assimilating new beliefs and exposing yourself to new experiences takes time and effort. It's about living by these newly accepted ideas while gently dismissing (ignoring) the ones that no longer serve you. Old patterns and mental habits may persist for a while as you begin this transformative process, and letting go of them is a vital part of your journey back to yourself. It's natural to experience discomfort during this period, as your conscious mind attempts to defend you by keeping you within familiar boundaries. Don't be discouraged or intimidated by this discomfort – it's simply part of the process.

Some people report feelings of sadness or frustration when they start to help themselves. This happens because your mind perceives change as unsafe at first and puts up defences. But those defences are temporary; with patience and persistence, your mind will adjust and feel secure in your new way of being.

Think of it as planting seeds and nurturing their growth. Many people lose patience and abandon the process too soon, assuming nothing is happening. But growth is happening, even if you can't yet see it. Beneath the surface, the seeds of your new ideas, beliefs and thoughts are germinating. Soon, if you hold on just a little longer, you'll see the seedlings emerge. Change takes time, but the blossoms will come – they always do.

This is a journey of becoming, not about 'fixing' an isolated part of you, such as your speech. Speech is an inseparable part of who you are, and as you grow and shift, the direction of your entire life shifts positively along with it.

Overcoming stuttering isn't about repairing a mechanical flaw within you by isolating and 'fixing' one malfunctioning part. Instead, it's a process that involves embracing your whole self – unpacking rather than suppressing. For the most dedicated individuals, this transformative process typically takes about eight months, although some may experience results sooner, as we've discussed earlier.

To make this return to your true self smoother and more enjoyable, I encourage you to embrace the concept of fun. Let this journey be light-hearted – don't take it too seriously. When you expect rapid results, it's easy to become overly focused on the final destination, which can make it hard to keep things playful and joyful. Fun is about being present in the moment and savouring the process as it unfolds, day by day. Constantly fixating on the outcome or 'watching the clock' drains the joy from the experience and adds unnecessary stress. And when rigid expectations and deadlines fuel stress, discomfort often follows, leading to resistance, disengagement and a sense of struggle.

It's important to remember that we naturally move towards what feels good and away from what feels uncomfortable. So, make every moment count. Focus on the process, not the outcome. Your path towards fluency and self-discovery is made up of countless small, daily steps (i.e. decisions, choices). The quality of these steps determines the quality of your destination. Prioritize the journey – the daily experiences – over the end result.

Be cautious of those who promise quick fixes. They're often charlatans preying on people's hopes and naivety. The process of dissolving speech anxiety requires a gradual 'unpacking' of your mind and personality. By gradual, I mean about a year of consistent practice and engagement. You may wonder, '*What if it's too hard for me to focus on the process and make it fun? What if I want fluency too much?*'

My answer is simple: you'll need to learn the art of letting go and trusting the process. This is your inner world, and only you can transform it. No one else can do it for you. As you progress, even small positive shifts in your emotions and their impact on your speech will build your confidence. This growing confidence will fuel your motivation to keep going.

Remember, the journey to the top of Everest is made one step at a time; no one runs to the summit in a flash. The ascent itself – the challenges, the growth, the transformation – is what makes the experience meaningful and deeply rewarding.

'I didn't just get lucky, nor did I discover a unique method of overcoming stuttering that works only for me. The difference between fluency and stuttering is rooted in our beliefs and perceptions – it's all about mindset.'

— Olga Bednarski

Reason 9: Pride and holding on to grudges. 'Nobody and nothing can ever help me.'

A belief that many PWS share is the conviction that 'nobody and nothing can help me'. The idea that 'my situation is so unique, so hopeless, that I'm beyond help' is often rooted in the pride of a wounded ego – a defence mechanism rejecting the possibility of assistance. This attitude frequently stems from earlier traumas, particularly when trust was betrayed by those you depended on during childhood or adolescence.

When trust is broken, it can lead to deep resentment, mistrust and even anger – towards others and the world at large. This betrayal makes it incredibly difficult to open up to anyone or to ask for and accept help, even when it's needed the most. Those who have experienced such pain often shut down, convinced that reaching out is futile. In my work, I've noticed that many individuals carry this guardedness into our first sessions. There's a noticeable distance, and the process of opening up – emotionally and mentally – feels almost insurmountable for them at first.

To truly receive help and support, you need to be open and willing to trust again. This can feel like an enormous challenge. The instinct to close yourself off – like a tightly sealed shell on a beach – is a natural defence. It's a way of protecting yourself from the risk of being hurt again. Building walls around yourself feels safer than risking rejection or betrayal by being vulnerable.

Hyper-independence often plays a role here, too. You might believe you can and must do everything alone, without any external support. This 'superhuman' mindset often arises from the painful belief that 'I'm alone' or 'I'm different from everyone else, so I can't rely on anyone'. For children who couldn't depend on their parents or caregivers, there's often a compulsion to grow up too quickly and appear unshakably strong. But this strength can be fragile. Beneath the mask of hyper self-reliance and independence, there's often a profound sense of loneliness and longing for connection.

The pride of a wounded ego is a significant barrier to seeking help – even when help is freely available. You may become overly suspicious, assuming there are charlatans or hidden motives behind every offer of assistance. This suspicion can lead to a sense of hopelessness or resignation, sometimes even before giving therapy or guidance a fair chance. It's essential to understand that your expectations play a pivotal role – they shape what you allow yourself to receive.

It's also important to consider that speaking – sharing your voice – is more than just opening your mouth. It's an act of vulnerability, of opening your mind and heart. Every time you share your thoughts, you expose yourself to the possibility of being accepted or rejected, judged or laughed at, applauded or ignored. The unpredictability of these outcomes requires trust – trust in yourself and in others. It requires courage to be vulnerable and to believe that, even if the world doesn't always respond kindly, you're still worthy of being heard.

For many PWS, the act of opening up and asking for help can be an obstacle. Often, they hide behind logical justifications for why they do not seek the support they need. These justifications become yet another defence mechanism, a shield crafted to protect themselves from the possibility of betrayal or hurt. However, this rationalization also keeps them disconnected from their authentic selves, preventing them from experiencing the deep, genuine self-acceptance they long for – not the kind imposed by societal norms, but a true acceptance born from within.

The path to overcoming this inner barrier begins with a conscious decision to open up, to allow love, support and help to flow into your heart, and to let go of resentment. This process involves a courageous willingness to take emotional risks, embracing the possibility of external reactions – or even silence – that might accompany your vulnerability.

Reason 10: Staying curious. Choosing simplicity over complexity. The art of inquiry.

One of the main reasons people fail to achieve the results they hope for is a deeply ingrained tendency to complicate things that are, at their core, simple. I realize that simplicity is a recurring theme in my writing. I'm here to reflect reality, not to sugar-coat it. When faced with a challenge – like stuttering – many people immediately focus on its perceived difficulty (i.e. external symptoms), bypassing the simplest and most obvious solutions and methods. We've been conditioned to believe that solving any 'problem' must involve a complex, arduous process. However, problems often begin to dissolve when we stop insisting they're complex and instead allow ourselves to see them through the lens of simplicity.

This tendency to overcomplicate often leads people into convoluted debates about stuttering, ranging from theories that it's a form of schizophrenia or Tourette's syndrome to claims that it's an unchangeable genetic condition. These debates, while passionate, rarely yield useful insights or solutions. Instead, they create division and resentment within the PWS community, driving people further away from meaningful progress.

The futility of these debates is plain to see: if there's no tangible improvement – if anxiety, discomfort and lost opportunities remain – then the issue persists. This is a clear signal that the path being pursued is not working, and these debates, no matter how engaging, ultimately lead nowhere.

Many of these discussions also point to external causes of stuttering – factors over which we seemingly have no control. Because this view is widely accepted, it often reinforces a sense of helplessness among PWS, making them feel like victims of an uncontrollable condition that 'just happens'. This belief can lead to despair, hopelessness and even anger, creating a divide between 'us' (PWS) and 'them' (society). Tragically, in some cases, it can lead to thoughts of self-harm or suicide – a heart-breaking reality, especially when help and solutions are available.

The solution lies right here, within your own mind. The mind created the problem, and it's the mind – once you learn to guide and nurture it – that will set your voice free. It's as simple as that.

When people ask me, '*How did you improve and overcome your stuttering?*' my answer is always this: '*I transformed my relationship with myself, and through that, my relationship with others and the world.*'

It all started with my willingness to experiment with my mental and emotional states. I began noticing that my speech was profoundly influenced by how I felt in different situations and around various people. In some circumstances, and with certain individuals, I felt calm, safe, present, physically relaxed and emotionally steady. These feelings created the conditions for my speech to flow naturally – without interruptions, without struggle. My whole being – mind, body and emotional state – aligned effortlessly to support ease and fluency.

As I spoke and engaged with others in this state, the positive experiences I was having reinforced themselves. Each pleasant interaction fed into the next, creating a self-sustaining cycle of confidence and joy.

Conversely, when I felt anxious, foggy-headed, physically tense or mentally scattered – caught in a web of overthinking – my speech instantly reflected that inner state. My breathing would become shallow, the flow of my words disrupted, leading to silent blocks and an uphill struggle. In these moments, my whole being aligned with tension and resistance. Each painful or frustrating interaction fuelled a cycle of negativity, amplifying my stress and reinforcing the very struggles I was trying to escape.

Over time, my personal observations were validated by others. More than 280 individuals – and counting – have shared their stories with me, recounting experiences that mirrored my own.

I believe we all have the capacity to observe – provided we consciously choose to slow down and pay attention. This means quieting that internal, argumentative voice that often tries to dismiss simplicity, urging us to dive headfirst into the murky waters of complexity – and, by default, unconsciousness (unawareness). Complexity is often glorified as 'the only right path' to finding answers, but it's also a path fraught with unnecessary suffering and delays. The truth is, you do not have to overcomplicate things. Let others run their marathon of overthinking while you choose to pause, soften the noise in your mind (often echoing the voices of others) and observe yourself with patience, compassion and understanding.

When you embrace this purposeful, mindful self-observation, the intricate dynamics of your speech anxiety will begin to reveal themselves. Your feelings will act as gentle guides, pointing you towards the unhelpful and often critical inner dialogues and stories that may be holding you back.

A loving reminder here: be intentional about what you seek during this self-exploration. If you allow yourself to be swayed by the socially accepted 'dis-ease model' and focus solely on the surface aspects of speech, you may find yourself stuck in a frustrating cycle, unable to move forward. Instead, set your intention to look beyond just speech. Dive deeper into your overall emotional state and how it influences your being – how it either nurtures a sense of flow or creates blockages.

When emotions and stories inevitably arise – and they will – meet them with kindness, not criticism. Resist the urge to judge yourself for what you think or feel. Instead, nurture curiosity. Why do you feel this way? Why are you telling yourself this particular story? Who might have first told it to you? Most importantly, could you choose a different narrative? One that uplifts you, rather than weighing you down or trapping you in an emotional rut?

Before moving on to answer your questions, I want to leave you with one final thought: learn to embrace and accept every step of this journey, letting go of obsessing over the final outcome. When you focus on waiting for results – whether by watching the clock or anxiously anticipating a breakthrough – you're not truly present in the process. And without presence, you can't engage. The transformation you seek comes from staying actively involved in the journey itself. It's the doing that brings about change.

Remember, the quality of your present moments – those small, meaningful steps – determines the quality of your future outcomes.

In the following sections, I'll address your questions and shine a light on the psychological and physical processes underlying verbal blocking and turbulence. Together, we'll explore these hidden mechanisms with clarity and compassion.

Questions & Answers

Understanding speech anxiety and stuttering

'I have no intention of telling you anything new; however, I want you to hear something new and say it to yourself. Repeatedly.'

— Olga Bednarski

Question 1:

I've read John Harrison's book *Redefining Stuttering* multiple times and deeply resonate with its message. However, while the ideas in the book are thought-provoking, they are just that – ideas. There are no specific techniques offered on how to achieve the freedom it describes. So, what do you do next?

A: One fresh, well-defined alternative idea – or, rather, a collection of ideas – is all you need to initiate a tremendous transformation and elevate your life to new heights. These collections of ideas form into ideologies, mental frameworks, belief systems or philosophies. Call them whatever resonates with you. Once accepted as your truths, they become guiding principles that shape your experiences, including how you perceive and approach speaking.

If you're currently struggling with anxiety, panic attacks, irrational fear or stuttering, it's a sign that the ideas you currently hold about yourself, others and life are not serving you. In fact, your current belief system may be working against the very things you long for: peace, quiet confidence, presence, good mental health, flow and a sense of ease and good fortune across all areas of life.

The concepts I share in this book are not limited to one area – they can be applied to nearly every aspect of your life. We live in a world of ideas. These ideologies, whether we consciously recognize them or not, influence our actions, behaviours and daily choices. Ultimately, they shape the experiences we have, whether that means living in a state of debilitating anxiety and fear or feeling a deep sense of peace and assurance that life, despite its occasional challenges, is always supporting and looking out for us.

What we often label as 'luck' is not luck at all. It's the result of aligning yourself with empowering new ideas – an ideology or philosophy of life. These ideas can be conscious or unconscious, but there's no mystery or magic involved. Once you're introduced to the right set of principles, the key is to live and act in alignment with them consistently. Over time – typically within three to eight months – these new ideas become part of your subconscious, automatically guiding your thoughts, actions and decisions effortlessly, much like learning to drive a car or swim.

Ideologies shape what we do, how we do it and even what we choose not to do it, ultimately determining the outcomes we experience and the fulfilment of our purpose. We live in the world of ideas – some trivial, others profound, both individual and societal. Your personal ideology defines the quality of every aspect of your life: your relationships, career choices, where you live, your aspirations, ambitions, how you set boundaries, the clothes you wear, your health, your self-care and beyond. In essence, ideas write the story of your life.

Even if you're unaware of it, your life is directed by a collection of ideas. These ideas play out in your reality daily, creating or manifesting the experiences you encounter. On a broader scale, societal ideologies – movements like environmentalism, body positivity, democracy or communism – shape the world around us. And yes, stuttering, too, is driven by an ideology: the way you relate to yourself, others and the world. Every ideology exists to fulfil a specific goal or lead to a clearly defined outcome.

Stuttering is sustained by a deeply personal collection of ideas – your mindset, your inner belief system – that keeps it firmly in place. My hope is that these words find someone ready to understand this issue at its core and see it for what it truly is.

Old, stagnant and fallacious ideas are like invasive weeds in an untended garden. What beauty can grow in a garden overrun with neglect? Very little. These stagnant ideas create struggle and suffering. The process of dissolving stuttering is like tending to your inner garden – removing the weeds of harmful, restrictive ideas and planting seeds of fresh, empowering thoughts.

Your most powerful tool for identifying and removing mental weeds is intentional observation – the ability to pay attention on purpose. Observation acts like a light in the impenetrable darkness of falsehood and anchors you to the 'now', bringing you presence and inner stillness. This allows you to step back (detach) from mind-created problems, so they lose their grip on you.

This tool, though simple, is often overlooked. Through observation, you train your mind to adopt a more detached perspective – a bird's-eye view – where you no longer see yourself as your stuttering (or any other challenge).

You stop identifying with it and defining yourself by it. Even if this separation lasts just a moment, it's enough to let you glimpse your true self – so much more than any predicament.

The process of dissolving stuttering is gradual, but even removing a single mental weed and replacing it with a healthy new idea can bring immediate and noticeable relief. That sense of relief you feel when a fresh idea takes root in your mind is a sign you're on the right path.

Ideas are incredibly powerful. They're contagious. Once planted, they can grow into fragrant flowers or invasive weeds. They can enslave or liberate, cripple or heal. Be intentional about the ideas you expose yourself to and nurture the empowering ones with care. This is what I call 'knowledge therapy'. By embracing these principles, you can cultivate the beautiful garden of your life – your own Garden of Eden. And it's already within you, waiting to flourish.

Don't dwell on your past. It defines you only as much as you allow it to. Most of us didn't grow up with healthy philosophies of life, but that doesn't have to hold us back. As adults, we have the gift of choice – and thanks to the brain's remarkable plasticity, change is always possible. Choose your ideology, live by its principles and the transformation you desire will come, often more swiftly than you imagine.

New ideas. Application. Consistency. Repetition. These are the keys to creating change – a lasting change.

You're the one who will go through this journey, and my objective is to make your path as clear and understandable as possible.

Watch extensive conversations with John Harrison on YouTube channel: Stop Stuttering with Olga

Question 2:

When you're cheerful, you tend to stutter more because you speak more, making the stuttering more noticeable. Conversely, when you're serious and quiet, you also stutter more due to speaking less. What exactly does stutter demand from us?

A: When you speak more, it often happens because you feel emotional or excited about something – perhaps cheerful and ecstatic. For PWS, these psychological states can trigger a subtle concern about coming across as 'too much' – too emotional, too eager, or over the top – even when the situation fully warrants such enthusiasm, like during an exhilarating moment such as bungee jumping. Without realizing it, the individual begins to 'put a lid on' their emotional expression. This behaviour (mostly unconscious and automatic) translates into holding back – an internal resistance to letting go.

Some PWS might perceive emotional displays as inappropriate, especially if they were raised with beliefs like 'children should be seen but not heard'. In such environments, expressing anger – or even joy – might have provoked parental disapproval or punishment. These early experiences can deeply shape how emotions are managed, often leading to suppression and a fear of fully expressing oneself.

When a person is serious and quiet, it can be helpful to examine the thoughts swirling in their mind during those moments. Typically, for PWS, their inner dialogue revolves around their speaking performance or speech-related aspects of their identity. This mental preoccupation often stirs up nervousness and discomfort, rooted in the fear of disappointing others or not measuring up. This psychological tension can begin long before a speaking situation arises, intensifying as the moment approaches and manifesting as physical discomfort – holding one's breath, tightness in the throat, or other sensations of tension. If this cycle isn't noticed and interrupted early, blocking becomes almost inevitable.

It's also worth considering the context of the situation in which resistance (both mental and physical) and stuttering occur – like a job interview or a group conversation. Just as in the example of cheerful excitement, here seriousness or quietness might mask intense emotions such as resentment, anger or discontent. Depending on their intensity, these emotions can be challenging to suppress – like bubbles in a shaken bottle of champagne. Yet, many PWS attempt to forcefully contain these feelings, fearing an 'ugly display' of emotion that might lead to rejection or accusations of being a troublemaker. This fear often stems from the shame or guilt they anticipate feeling afterwards, even when their feelings are entirely reasonable or justified, such as in cases of a legitimate grievance or violation of personal boundaries.

Ironically, the harder one tries to suppress or control emotions, the more powerful and overwhelming they become. Compulsion to control amplifies negative emotions. Suppression, in essence, is holding back. This mental effort creates physical consequences – glottal tension, muscular spasms and the associated difficulties with speaking.

So, what does stuttering demands from us? I wouldn't use the word 'demand'. Instead, I would say it nudges us towards letting go and expressing ourselves rather than repressing our emotions. It's as if stuttering is showing you the way – urging you to release control and step out of your own way. Physically, there's no obstacle preventing the normal flow of speech. The invisible, yet very real, obstacle is in the mind, which prevents you from feeling safe enough to be your authentic self. This heightened self-consciousness and compulsion to control – designed to ensure safety – ultimately blocks your natural expression.

You can begin to move past this by re-examining your relationship with yourself, other people and the world around you. As your beliefs, ideas and perceptions shift, your need to control will ease, as will the mental habits and micro-behaviours associated with it – like holding your breath or rehearsing mentally. As you cultivate a sense of inner safety, trust and comfort, your body will naturally loosen, creating space for speech to flow freely.

Question 3:

What are the psychological aspects of my blocking?

A: The most prominent factor contributing to blocking is the emotional or psychological discomfort an individual experiences in the presence of certain people or in specific situations. Often, this discomfort begins long before the actual event or interaction takes place. It builds up over time, becoming stronger – and sometimes more debilitating – as the social event approaches.

This emotional discomfort sets in motion what John Harrison refers to as the phenomenon of holding back. Holding back can also be described as compulsive control, inner tension, pressure or resistance – different terms for the same experience. It arises as a protective mechanism, designed to prevent an individual from engaging in an activity (in this case, speaking) due to perceived conscious or unconscious threats, such as fear, shame or guilt. Put simply, this resistance acts as a shield, trying to protect you from the pain of a perceived 'social failure' and the torrent of overwhelming emotions that might follow.

Many PWS attempt to manage this inner discomfort by engaging in behaviours I've described as the 'Multiple Task Paradigm' in my first book, *The Anatomy of Stuttering* (Bednarski, 2022). This phenomenon involves trying to consciously control and monitor every detail of their inner experience, the speech-motor system and the social interaction – all at the same time. While it may provide the illusion of control, in reality this multitasking creates mental overwhelm. Instead of reducing discomfort, it increases the likelihood of disrupted social performance.

When this happens, the aftermath can be excruciating. Many PWS replay the situation repeatedly in their minds, accompanied by harsh self-criticism. This self-abusive rhetoric amplifies anxiety and reinforces the problem, creating a vicious cycle that can feel impossible to escape – until it's recognized for what it is. Becoming aware of these patterns is the first major step towards making speaking less intimidating, strengthening your emotional well-being, and making life feel lighter and easier.

The push-and-pull effect

Holding back is often experienced as a 'push-and-pull' dynamic: on one hand, you deeply want to talk, to express yourself freely. But on the other hand, the inner discomfort is so strong that it pulls you back, putting a lid on your expression. This inner conflict can lead to staying silent – or struggling through turbulence when you do speak.

As humans, we instinctively steer away from discomfort and towards comfort. When you feel at ease, you're naturally motivated to speak, to let go and to flow. Remember those fleeting moments of fluency, where words seemed to come effortlessly? That's the flow I'm talking about – the feeling of driving without a handbrake on.

Before you can achieve that flow, however, it's essential to address the mental resistance that holds you back. Keep reading to learn how – or perhaps you haven't already figured it out.

Question 4:

You'll find it has never been your stutter getting in the way of you living life, but instead your anxiety and lack of confidence. Is this possible?

A: Absolutely! That, along with how you acted, behaved and responded due to anxiety and a lack of confidence, plays a significant role. Anxiety and low confidence are fuelled by your thoughts and inner narratives – they shape your inner climate, your overall state of being.

When you begin to shift those thoughts and replace them with more life-affirming ones, the way you feel about yourself will naturally transform. You'll approach situations with a renewed attitude, feeling lighter and more open. As a result, the experiences that once filled you with dread and trepidation will carry less tension and holding back. Instead, you'll navigate them with greater ease, freedom and even enjoyment.

Question 5:

My ten-year-old son stutters. When you were young, what are one or two key things you wish people understood, and what do you wish they would stop doing?

A: I truly wish there was more understanding of what speech anxiety is all about, along with greater support for people like me in the form of patience, kindness and genuine human empathy from educators. I also wish there was more education for parents – and for myself as well. If I had access to even a fraction of the information I know now, it would have brought so much relief. I wouldn't have felt 'less than' or inferior, and my self-esteem wouldn't have suffered as much.

When my stuttering first developed, I didn't know how to understand it or how to manage the overwhelming anxiety that consumed me on a daily basis. I wish there had been more education about speech anxiety and its underlying causes. This is part of why I've written this book: to help shed light on this topic and offer others the knowledge and understanding I lacked.

Question 6:

My son struggles with breathing properly while speaking. We've tried singing lessons without success. He used to hold his breath and rush through sentences, but now he's making some noises. I'm not sure if these are habits or tics. Can you suggest any strategies to help him break these habits?

A: From what you've described, it sounds like your son is experiencing anxiety, which manifests as holding his breath and rushing through sentences. Breathing is deeply connected to how we speak – it's impossible to speak without full, regular breathing. Stuttering begins in the mind and is then expressed as verbal blocks and stuttered speech. Essentially, speaking is the invisible behaviour that becomes visible when stuttering occurs. Holding back breath is often an attempt to suppress uncomfortable or frightening feelings in order to avoid being overwhelmed.

I'm not sure how old your son is or how long these tics and habits have been present, but, if I were you, I wouldn't immediately label them as stuttering. Instead, I would recommend taking a step back and assessing your child's emotional health and how he typically deals with his feelings. How are emotions handled in your family? Are they expressed openly, or are they repressed? How do you personally deal with both positive and negative emotions? Has your child ever seen you cry? Is there room in your home to talk about feelings, or are they often brushed aside and deemed irrelevant or inappropriate? Children learn from the adults around them and often adopt our coping mechanisms without questioning whether these strategies are helpful or not. This kind of review of your family's emotional well-being would be a great starting point.

If you notice areas where improvement is needed – for example, if emotions are dismissed as unimportant – perhaps it would be helpful to change this routine. Invite your child into a more open dialogue but lead by example. It's important to invite conversation, but not to push too hard. Let your child know you're here for them if they want to talk, and give them space when they need it.

How long have you been trying singing as a technique? It's essential to remember that any exercise or technique takes time to have an effect and become more habitual. How long this takes will vary from person to person and will depend on the goals you're trying to achieve. Patience is key. Also, it's important to make sure that your child genuinely enjoys singing and is motivated to participate, rather than it being something solely driven by you. It's important to check in with their interests before signing them up for any classes.

The erratic breathing patterns and noises you mentioned (unless there are diagnosed physical causes) suggest to me that your son may be experiencing anxiety. I don't believe this is the same kind of stuttering that's seen in adults. Lastly, I would like to remind you that children's stuttering is often developmental and can be a temporary phase in speech development. Creating a safe, open and non-judgmental space for your child to discuss their emotions – and even for you as a parent to share your feelings – is crucial. Be patient as you begin this process, especially if this kind of communication is new to your family. It will take time to get comfortable with this new dynamic, but it will become a valuable part of your family life.

On a final note, I encourage you to look into selective mutism. While it may seem similar to stuttering, it's a condition that only occurs in certain situations and with specific people, typically those whom the child finds intimidating, such as teachers or authority figures. Sadly, parents can fall into this category as well, which is why I recommend reflecting on your relationship with your child. Selective mutism is a situational condition triggered by stress, where the vocal cords freeze, causing the person to stop speaking or breathe erratically. The symptoms usually fade once the trigger – such as an authority figure – leaves the situation.

Question 7:

When you focus all your time and energy on a clear goal or purpose, you may find less time to blame your stuttering or curse your luck. However, ensure that fluency itself isn't the goal. What are your thoughts on this?

A: This is the best and most effective strategy. Stuttering, like any challenge, is fuelled by the attention we give it. The more we think about it, blame it, resent it, fight it or agonize over it, the bigger it becomes – filling our mental space and becoming the centre of our existence. Attention is the fuel that energizes and reinforces stuttering.

So, what's the solution to this self-imposed struggle? The answer is simple yet profound: do the opposite. Intentionally turn your attention away from speech mechanics and focus it instead on your goals and purpose. Direct your mind towards something greater than speech itself – your dreams, plans and the life you want to create. Overwhelm your mind with positive, meaningful pursuits that inspire you, and let fluency become a natural by-product of this new state of being.

Our inner states – whether they are calm, anxious, kind or confident – always manifest in our bodies. Chasing after fluency or obsessing over it only amplifies the problem because fluency isn't something you can 'get' by force. It's the natural outcome of inner alignment and self-work.

You are doing an amazing job! Keep going – you're on the right path.

Question 8:

You've likely heard of people who overcome stuttering and speak freely. Since there's no guaranteed cure, how did they achieve this? We know that behavioural therapy alone isn't a magic solution.

A: Cure – a word that suggests stuttering is a disease. But it's not. Many have 'recovered' or gone into 'remission' without medical intervention. Words matter. They shape your attitudes, actions and outcomes. For instance, if you believe stuttering is an incurable genetic disorder, how can you hope to move forward, let alone succeed? Highly unlikely.

Those who have succeeded from the outset refused to abide by the so-called 'rule' that stuttering is incurable. They sought solutions in uncharted territories. From my own journey, I can tell you this: I never accepted the notion that stuttering was a permanent condition. Information to the contrary simply passed me by, unabsorbed. My path began with curiosity – questions that demanded answers – and strategies that carried me ever closer to freedom. I ignored everything, no matter how scientific, that contradicted my objective: overcoming anxiety and blocking. My experience had already shown me fluent speech was possible. I focused on finding, applying and refining the tools that would lead me to my goal.

At that time, desperation fuelled me. I couldn't afford to wallow in the problem or linger in acceptance as some do. I needed a practical, workable solution – and fast. And so, I found it.

Stepping away from commonly accepted notions, even those rooted in science, is essential if you're seeking true progress. Extraordinary results demand an extraordinary approach. You can't achieve freedom while marching to the same lulling tune repeated to the majority.

My path wasn't about one miraculous method but a blend of approaches. I used techniques like cognitive-behavioural therapy and self-hypnosis and invented others as I progressed. Intuition guided me. Each success became a steppingstone towards freedom. Alongside these techniques, I experienced transformative insights – moments that shifted my perspective, particularly regarding emotional challenges and how they can be resolved without endlessly unpacking personal history.

When I began this journey, I had no guide. There was no John Harrison or anyone like him in my awareness. I walked alone. It was trial and error – a game of discovery. Each step taught me something new, and I continue to learn as I walk this path of self-discovery. To find freedom, I had to look beyond the obvious, past stuttering and the noise of widely accepted ideas, and question everything. Only then could I find my way.

Many people rely heavily on the words of 'authorities', seldom questioning their credibility or motives. The more authoritative the source, the more unquestionable it seems. But what if you embarked on your own investigation? What if you drew from your experiences and those of people who have succeeded? Why cling to communities that fail to progress, where misery becomes a shared currency?

You have a choice. This is your life.

Sadly, in many stuttering communities, advancement of understanding is stifled. Any glimmer of light or independent thought is quickly snuffed out. This suppression feels purposeful – an effort to keep people from asking questions like, 'How do others succeed?' Once curiosity ignites, change becomes inevitable. Independence threatens the structures that rely on keeping people tethered to the problem. After all, if you found freedom, the system wouldn't be necessary.

Having spoken to hundreds of PWS, I can confidently say this: the knowledge you need to set yourself free is all around you. You can do this alone. But – and this is critical – you must first see the knowledge and apply it. To do so, you need to shift your focus away from the distractions of limiting beliefs and open your eyes to another way. Once you see that way, pursue it with all your heart. That is how you awaken from the deep slumber of unawareness.

You might think you're tackling stuttering, but the truth is deeper. What you're challenging is a system – a matrix – designed to keep you disconnected from yourself, scared and therefore easily controlled. This is achieved by destabilizing mental health, first by provoking issues, then ensuring they persist for life.

What you're overcoming are malfunctioning mental programs (or, mental habits) manifesting as stuttering or speech anxiety. By reconnecting with your inner power and vitality, you rediscover the person you were meant to be – fear free.

Where others see only speech issues, I saw connections. Thoughts, beliefs, perceptions, attitudes, personality, mental clutter – all these elements influence our ability to express ourselves.

If even one person has found freedom, it's proof that you can too.

Question 9:

Could you explain the link between cognitive thought disorder, psychosis and stuttering?

A: All mind-created (mindset-driven) challenges can, over time, contribute to the development of a psychotic personality or other comorbid psychological conditions. Some of these issues can be effectively managed through mindset work alone, while others may be more severe and require a combination of approaches. For instance, pharmacological treatment might be needed alongside cognitive-behavioural therapy, mindfulness practices, emotional regulation techniques, or other supportive methods tailored to the individual and their preferences.

In the case of speech anxiety, it's important to recognize that it may sometimes be heightened by an underlying or coexisting condition, particularly if that condition is left untreated or goes unnoticed.

Question 10:

I was recently diagnosed with cluttering disorder, and the doctor said I have a combination of cluttering and slight stuttering. My cluttering is severe compared to my stuttering, and I speak incredibly fast, causing me to skip words, letters and syllables. Is it possible to overcome or control this problem?

A: These are emotional challenges at their core driven and propelled by cluttered (negatively conditioned) mind. To overcome your difficulties, it's essential to address and heal the underlying emotional causes. It's frustrating how institutions create various labels and definitions that don't actually explain anything, nor do they provide any real relief or guidance on how to ease the symptoms. Speaking 'incredibly fast', for example, is often a sign of high anxiety originating from negative conditioning. I've even encountered fluent speakers who do the same.

My suggestion to you is to set aside these labels for now, and instead begin exploring your inner world. Start addressing what truly needs attention – whether it's 'recovering from your childhood', engaging in self-inquiry or anything else that might bring healing. Take full responsibility for your life and its direction. Intentionally choose your thoughts. Take control of your life and steer it in the direction you want to go. Remember, unless you change, nothing changes.

De-clutter.

Question 11:

If stuttering was easy to overcome, do not you think that people would have already known about it? If so, why don't we still?

A: The solution to stuttering is simple and straightforward, but it requires being alert, awake and present. One must detach from the mind-created drama and the endless games surrounding the problem to clearly see how it all works. Unfortunately, the majority of people – not just those who stutter – are deeply unconscious, caught in a kind of mental slumber. They remain fully identified with their internal drama and predicaments that arise from it, whether it's stuttering, anxiety, depression, addiction, marital struggles or other challenges. This immersion blinds them to the true causes of their problems, leaving them unable to see a way out.

To break free from this identification with the mind, one must cultivate sharp awareness and stillness. It's a skill, not a pill. With time, dedication and staying on track, clarity emerges. Gradually, it becomes self-evident how the mind's narratives have been blocking the path forward. It's as if the road, once strewn with obstacles, suddenly clears, allowing unhindered movement. The answers have always been there – they're not hidden – but recognizing them is a challenge for an untrained and cluttered mind. This is why so many remain stuck in a cycle of confusion and 'paradigm paralysis'.

Even science isn't immune to paradigm paralysis. Once a theory is proposed, it's often declared 'truth' and defended stubbornly, even when it no longer serves. Revisions are slow to come, and progress stagnates. This is precisely what has happened with stuttering. Until people start questioning outdated models and shifting their understanding, the delay in finding a workable, widely accessible solution will persist – potentially for decades more. Waiting for institutions to provide the answers is a futile exercise; the power lies with each individual.

Many people around the world are already beginning to see the true causes of speech anxiety and are successfully overcoming it.

Question 12:

Can you explain why people who stutter speak fluently for the first few minutes after waking up?

A: When you first wake up, your mind hasn't yet had the chance to fall back into its usual 'course of action' – holding back or stuttering. In those early moments, you're in a different state of consciousness. Your brain is still producing theta waves, which are associated with relaxation, introspection and subconscious activity.

As you move through your day, however, your brain shifts to producing beta waves. These are linked to active thinking, problem-solving and alertness. Since stuttering is a mind-created issue, the act of thinking about or remembering it activates the habitual patterns of holding back and resistance. This, in turn, leads to the predictable result: stuttered speech.

I encourage you to explore my insights on how cannabis, alcohol and other stimulants can similarly trigger temporary 'remission' and why that happens. Ultimately, the principle remains the same: less thinking, more presence, less or no stuttering.

Question 13:

Why does my speech improve when I am tired, or ill?

'Tiredness is a gift that allows us to finally understand and experience what surrender, and non-resistance truly feel like.'

— Olga Bednarski

A: When you're ill or tired, you enter an altered state of consciousness. The habitual state we live in daily, often on autopilot, begins to lose its grip. The conditioned mind, with its predictable behaviours, starts to lose its hold on the body, and suddenly we feel free from anxiety and stuttering. Our usual mental activity slows down. Simply put, we forget to stutter for a brief period, as stuttering is no longer the central focus of our attention and gets pushed aside. When we no longer give it our attention, the problem fades away. This often happens in the morning, too – when you wake up, refreshed and just emerging from the world of dreams. Your mind forgets to stutter and you're granted a brief period of flow. However, after a while, the mind remembers its old patterns and begins to replay the same 'old track'.

When we're tired or ill, we become liberated from the stream of thinking about our problematic speech. This is why, unexpectedly, stuttering stops. It shows us that stuttering is a problem created and fuelled by the mind – and nothing else. When the mind is distracted or forgets to worry about speech, we are free. Once the tiredness or illness subsides, the mind remembers it's supposed to worry about speech again, and stuttering returns.

The incessant stream of thinking must stop. When the mind becomes quiet, the problems disappear. However, when the mind re-engages, the old problems resurface. When the mind stops, you're free from the problem of stuttering and the identity that comes with it. The real, fluent you comes to the front. The problem only exists in the mind because it was created by the mind.

This same thing happens in emergency situations, when the mind doesn't have time to dwell on the stuttering story. In these moments, stuttering is no longer on the agenda. The mind stops, you become fully present in the now, and something more powerful takes over as you handle the situation, and stuttering evaporates.

If you don't remember the problem, it's gone.

Question 14:

Is there a stuttering gene?

A: There's no such thing as a 'stuttering gene'. The only genetic factor in speech anxiety is the type of nervous system a person has, or their natural temperament. Some children are simply more sensitive or impressionable than others.

Other children, for example, may develop different issues, like toilet anxiety or incontinence. What develops depends on a variety of factors – circumstances, parenting style and how the child reacts to and interprets their experiences.

If you have family members who stutter, this doesn't mean you have a 'stuttering gene'. It's more likely that these family members were exposed to similar environmental factors and had similar experiences. For example, emotionally cold or harsh treatment, neurotic mothers or being expected to grow up quickly and take on adult responsibilities – sometimes even parenting their own parents – could all contribute to the development of speech anxiety. These shared experiences trigger similar responses. I've shared some general examples here, but you can reflect on your own experiences to fill in the gaps and understand where this 'family gene' actually comes from.

Also, keep in mind that a child's experiences don't have to be extremely dramatic (e.g. trauma like abuse or neglect) to have an impact. It's not the event itself that causes trauma, but how a child interprets it and how it integrates with their worldview. I've heard of cases where the death of a pet, coupled with a dismissive attitude from a parent, was enough to trigger initial distress – distress that, as a child, was misinterpreted. What follows is a process of learning and reinforcement, which ultimately solidifies as anxiety around speaking.

In the end, it's the environment that activates the 'gene'. Genes do not activate on their own.

Question 15:

How can you explain the research findings that prove existence of the stuttering gene?

A: The moment I learned that researchers were using mice as subjects in studies about the causes of stuttering in humans, it completely discredited the whole thing for me. Animals do not possess the gift of speech, and therefore, logically, should never be used in such research. To me, this idea seems as absurd as it gets. However, it's worth noting that when humans are determined to find something, we become remarkably inventive in constructing evidence and even creating rational explanations to support it. These explanations may sound convincing, but only to an equally irrational, unconscious and deluded mind – much like the idea of 'stuttering mice'. With just a bit of critical and independent thinking, the delusions fall apart.

There's another type of brain study on those who stutter. What these studies reveal isn't the cause of stuttering, but the changes that result from living with speech anxiety, most likely over a prolonged period. Our brains are physically altered by our thoughts and habitual emotional states, and there's ample research supporting this. While science does uncover some truths, particularly in reference to brain scans, what these scans show is a tendency towards stuttering (such as heightened emotionality), not a 'stuttering gene', because no such thing exists.

Science often likes to label different forms of human suffering, package them up and then rest on its laurels by offering pills to ease the pain. I see a significant limitation in this approach. My mission is to offer people workable solutions, not just elaborate theories.

As a researcher, I can confidently say that science is not an exact science – there are exceptions where bias is reduced (such as in computational or observational studies), but it's never fully eliminated. Science is inevitably influenced by those who conduct it – by their perceptions, ideas, expectations and the culture in which they're embedded.

Don't accept everything you hear or read as the absolute truth. Choose your own truth, test it practically and adjust it as needed until you find what truly works and sustains you.

Question 16:

How do you define stuttering?

A: Stuttering isn't a neurological issue, but rather a reflection of personality – one shaped by a complex set of traits, beliefs, attitudes, perceptions and conditioned responses to events, situations and people. For most individuals without significant cognitive impairments, there's no organic or physical cause for stuttering.

The stuttering personality is built upon erroneous mental configurations – false, often toxic beliefs and ideas about oneself, others, situations, relationships and the world at large.

Once these limiting ideas are identified and replaced, the personality naturally begins to change as well. The person starts to feel safer in the world, much more comfortable in their own skin, expressing their thoughts freely without fear of judgment or criticism. They no longer depend on external validation or approval.

In essence, the person becomes unapologetically themselves, returning to their true authenticity. As a result, this opens the floodgates not only for speech but for all areas of life. Stuttering is fundamentally a problem of personality and has little to do with the physical act of speaking. Once the personality shifts, everything else follows.

Many so-called 'mysterious and unexplained' human struggles that were once dismissed as 'genetic' are driven by specific personality types. Take cancer, for instance – often referred to as the disease of 'good people' who chronically suppress their own needs and desires in order to help or save others, even to their own detriment. Research is already available on this phenomenon.

Obesity, too, is not a matter of neurology, thick bones or dieting; it's a problem of personality. And, just like stuttering, it can be reversed, helping individuals to reach and maintain healthy weight, if they choose to do so.

This is a deep and fascinating topic, and there's so much to explore.

Our personalities have the power to set the trajectory of our lives and shape our experiences – including the experience of speaking.

To underestimate the power of personality is to miss a key part of the human experience.

Question 17:

What has stuttering to do with driving and how to let go of control?

A: A bad driving experience (fear of driving) and a bad speaking experience (fear of speaking/stuttering) have a lot in common. It's only when you let go, stop overthinking, worrying and rehearsing, and trust in your ability to drive or speak, that the experience becomes effortless, enjoyable and even fun. Speaking is one of those experiences where *trying* to control everything actually ruins it – just like dancing, walking, or even sex. When you try to control it, you take away the joy, naturalness and spontaneity.

Question 18:

After all these years, what's the key aspect you learned about stuttering? What's at the core of this problem?

A: We're not truly overcoming anything except for our own cluttered, conditioned mind. What we're dealing with is a process of spiritual awakening, where stuttering (or any other emotional challenge) acts as a persistent distraction – a tricky, mind-made conundrum or game that keeps people preoccupied. It restrains personal growth and prevents us from reconnecting to our authenticity, which is a process of transcendence.

The severity of this preoccupation varies among individuals, but the essence remains the same. For some, the journey towards emancipation can be particularly challenging, leading to suffering and turmoil. This is why, I believe, it's urgent to educate people on how their minds work and teach emotional and mental regulation. In the work I do, I stand with those who are actively seeking answers, rather than waiting for institutions – who may take decades – to officially recognize and adopt alternative approaches to mental and physical well-being.

Everything I've mentioned is a skill that can be learned at any time with consistent practice and a willingness to embrace it.

Question 19:

Why there any times when I don't stutter?

A: Stuttering is a learned response, a reflection of the stuttering personality. But remember, your personality is simply an adaptation – a blend of your authentic traits and conditioned behaviours. Often, what we think of as our personality is a mix of genuine qualities and learned coping mechanisms, including those that don't align with our true nature, like stuttering (holding back).

Those fleeting moments of freedom you sometimes experience? They're not an illusion – they're glimpses of your personality letting go, releasing its grip and simply relaxing. In those moments, your genuine strengths, the core of who you truly are, begin to shine. They finally have the space to stretch out, grow and reveal themselves fully.

Question 20:

I stutter, even when I'm not anxious, why does it happen and how to prevent blocking?

A: Speech dynamics – the habitual actions you use to produce speech – can become misaligned, which is why stuttering occurs even when there's no anxiety or emotional overwhelm.

Stuttering is a learned response, where PWS have come to associate speaking with a strenuous, effortful experience. This creates a habitual pattern of pushing and fighting to get words out. This habit forms one of the key components of the dynamics of stuttering, alongside factors like breathing, attention, tempo, intention and underlying beliefs.

When you experience fluency, all these components work together in perfect harmony. It's like the engine of a car: when every part functions seamlessly, the car glides effortlessly down the road, and you, the driver, enjoy the ride. But when one or more parts of the engine falters or fails to perform, the ride becomes bumpy, stressful and uncertain. Instead of enjoying the journey, you're preoccupied with diagnosing the problem and worrying about breaking down.

To prevent blocking, it's essential to become consciously and acutely aware of how your habits contribute to the blocks. Once you identify what actions or patterns are unproductive, you can begin replacing them with behaviours that foster greater flow and ease.

Mindset and self-perception

'You are only as inferior as you think. Choose superior thoughts, and you will soar.'

— Olga Bednarski

Question 21:

How can I stop feeling inferior because of my stammer and stop putting others on a pedestal?

A: The short answer here would be: change your perspective and stop seeing yourself as inferior and others as superior.

How you think about yourself will inevitably shape how you feel, behave and the feedback you receive from others. Most PWS have a dysfunctional relationship with themselves, including a low self-opinion and negative self-judgment. What I've learned from my personal experience is that it doesn't matter if others criticise you, don't believe in you, or even hate you. What matters most is whether you criticise or support yourself. If, despite all the negativity from others, you choose to stand by your side, you will succeed because your core will remain intact and strong. But if you begin criticising yourself internally, this can lead to emotional, spiritual and. sadly, even physical self-destruction. So, dear reader, no matter what happens around you, you must build an internal fortress of unconditional support for yourself – one that can withstand all seasons and storms. Learn from your experiences, correct your mistakes as and when needed, while always being on your side. Always.

Pay attention to your inner dialogue, whether you're around people or alone. What do you typically say to yourself about yourself? What stories do you tell in your mind? For instance, if you spill a glass of red wine on the carpet or bump your elbow on the door frame, what do you say to yourself? How do you react? Do you hear name-calling?

Thoughts are incredibly powerful, and our habitual thoughts shape our personal experiences. This isn't esoteric; it's science, backed by solid evidence – the law of resonance. People use it to attract wealth, love and success in their lives, so why not use it to improve your speaking (or social experiences)?

The principle is the same. If you want to improve your social experiences, you simply need to adjust your internal variables accordingly.

Make a list of your typical responses – those habitual words you say to yourself in situations like the ones above. Now, how do you feel about yourself when you respond in such ways? Can you see the connection between your thoughts (your verbal responses) and your emotional state? If you feel angry, '*less than*', or disappointed with yourself, your behaviour will align with those negative thoughts and emotions. Whatever you believe about yourself will be confirmed through your experiences, creating a self-fulfilling prophecy, which only fuels a vicious cycle.

To break the cycle and improve the quality of your social experiences, you must first alter the quality of your internal emotional experiences – your inner weather. Stop putting yourself down, stop clipping your wings and start lifting yourself up. Understand and forgive yourself. Choose to see the greatness in you. This is how you cultivate self-love – a gift many PWS are severely lacking. Never criticize yourself. Instead, choose to understand and forgive.

We've been conditioned to believe that criticism leads to improvement and prevents mistakes. But no, my friend, you've been lied to. Where there is criticism, there is no learning, no growth. Mistakes are an essential part of learning. If you don't make mistakes – or if you're afraid to make them – you will not make any progress. You'll just keep procrastinating and postponing your life. The worst critic you can have is the one that lives in your head, and the most punishing voice is your own. Choose to be kind and compassionate with yourself. When you apply this simple concept, you'll find that instead of fearing new steps, you'll embrace curiosity, which makes you more willing to try and experiment. You'll let go of the need for perfection – because perfection and fear of failure are two sides of the same coin. This is where fun and progress truly begin!

Comparing yourself to others is always a losing, soul-destroying game. It's like chasing a horizontal line that moves further away as you approach it. It's pointless! Does it help you cultivate self-love and self-appreciation? No. If you must compare, compare yourself only to who you were yesterday, last week, last month or last year. Notice and appreciate your own progress.

Stop running the marathon of perfectionism. Slow down inside and take time to recognize and appreciate your progress. I know that many PWS (but this is true for everyone, not just PWS) get so caught up in their past that when change comes knocking, they ignore it, failing to notice their achievements. They constantly demand more perfection from themselves, which only leads to a sense of perpetual dissatisfaction – as if they're on a treadmill, never quite arriving. The more you try to be perfect, the less authentic you become. Perfection acts as a mask, a shield, a straitjacket that hides the real you. Deep down, you may have been made to believe that being real is unwelcome, embarrassing or punishable. So, you present an edited, stunted version of yourself to the world, fully convinced that this is what must be accepted. But nothing could be further from the truth.

Your self-consciousness and anxiety around people stem from idolizing them, believing they're perfect and you're defective. This belief fosters fear of rejection and causes you to hold back from opening up, preventing your natural, most authentic self from emerging. As I suspect, you may be engaging in a masquerade, trying to be someone else by playing different roles to fit in and be liked. The antidote to this is to stop idolizing others. Instead, look at people with curiosity and an open mind, seeing that they, too – whether fluent or not – have their own challenges.

PWS often become consumed by their speech, giving it so much attention that it fills their entire mental space, creating tunnel vision and restricting their view of all the other wonderful aspects of who they are. I dare you to look beyond your stuttering!

One final point, and this can be used as an exercise of self-discovery: see yourself as more than just a person who stutters. See yourself as the multidimensional, sentient being that you are. Your most powerful tools here are your curiosity, openness and self-observation. Don't underestimate yourself – there's so much you do not yet know about who you are.

Watch your negative self-talk. Notice your progress. Practise forgiveness and self-understanding. Don't idolize others. Study them, see them for who they are and recognize that you are more than your stutter. You're a multidimensional, sentient being.

Question 22:

Have you found any positive aspects of your stutter? For me, it's been a great 'asshole detector'. If someone is rude about my stutter or reacts negatively, I can dismiss them more quickly than those who don't stutter.

A: Stuttering often makes people more hypersensitive to even the smallest social cues, and it's common to interpret them negatively, even when no negativity is intended. Over time, we can develop a kind of working theory, believing that others are judging our speaking performance. The truth is, people do not judge your speech as much as you judge it yourself.

When you're constantly on the lookout for 'judgmental' people, you're more likely to find them. Many fluent speakers don't fully understand stuttering. They may have heard the word, but have never really observed it in action, so they don't always know what to expect or how to respond. I've heard many PWS mention feeling self-conscious when others laugh instinctively when they block, or when their face contorts during a block. But trust me, these reactions often come from confusion, not malice. At least, I like to believe that most people don't laugh intentionally.

It's also important to recognize that PWS can sometimes anticipate negative reactions from others based on past experiences, and we can interpret even the smallest facial expressions, a giggle or a lingering glance as hostile or judgmental. I encourage you to be mindful of these tendencies and try not to jump to negative conclusions about people who may not fully understand what you're going through when you block. If you do, you may find yourself becoming overly suspicious, paranoid and anxious. Give others some grace, especially when you're meeting them for the first time. If it helps, you can always share that you have a stutter before meeting.

A helpful practice I recommend before speaking events or meetings is asking yourself, 'What do I expect or anticipate from this situation with the people I'm about to meet? How do I want to be seen?' Imagine how you would like to be treated, how you want others to react to you, and how you would like to feel while speaking. Be as detailed as you like. Once you've done this, anticipate understanding, patience, meaningful conversations and genuine interest in you – and you'll likely find that you receive exactly that. This simple exercise is called modelling the situation, and it's an incredibly powerful tool.

Finally, once you reach a place of greater self-acceptance, negative reactions from others seem to diminish or even disappear. This happens because people reflect our perceptions of ourselves. When you shift your own expectations and view of yourself, the people around you'll often seem kinder and more accepting as well.

Question 23:

How do you handle the mental and emotional aspects of stuttering?

A: Begin by working with your thoughts and the underlying beliefs that shape them. If you're unsure which specific thoughts or beliefs lead to feelings of anxiety, irrational fear or excessive insecurity, try asking yourself this powerful question: 'What must I believe about myself to feel this way (e.g. anxious, fearful, insecure)?'

When you ask this question, resist the urge to overanalyse or rationalize intellectually. Instead, allow yourself to feel. Let the emotions surface naturally; these feelings will eventually transform into thoughts, providing valuable insight. This process allows you to connect with the deeper, subconscious beliefs driving your patterns, rather than just skimming the surface with conditioned reasoning. Through this, you'll begin to understand which inner beliefs lead you to think and feel the way you do consistently.

Once you identify these beliefs or inner narratives (writing them down is highly recommended), you can begin the process of challenging them. This is not something that happens all at once – it's a journey. As you progress, a fuller picture will gradually emerge.

Approach this work with lightness and curiosity. Play a mental game of call and response, making it as engaging and fun as possible. Avoid falling into seriousness or rigidity. For instance, you might hold a belief like, 'People judge me solely based on my speech.' Challenge this thought: 'Is that true? Is that really all people see in me? Isn't there so much more to who I am?' Shift your focus away from stuttering as the centrepiece of your attention and life. Intentionally broaden your perspective, stepping outside the repetitive and often limiting thought patterns surrounding it.

As you shift the meaning you attach to social situations, you'll find greater ease and confidence in these moments. What new belief could serve you better, improving both your interactions and your emotional well-being? Perhaps something like: 'There is so much more to me than my speech, and people are willing to see and appreciate that.'

Say this to yourself often and notice how it changes your inner state. It can take you from anxiety or guilt to self-compassion, curiosity and peace of mind. Over time, this new belief will naturally influence your behaviour, leading to changes in your reality and the way others respond to you. The transformation is inevitable!

Mastering self-control over your thoughts and emotions is one of the greatest achievements you can strive for – and it's absolutely within your reach.

'When studying stuttering through the real-life experiences of people who stutter, it becomes impossible not to see the true source of the problem – the human mind.'

— Olga Bednarski

Question 24:

Can stuttering lead to becoming mute? This thought has been on my mind. I always believed my stuttering would improve with age, but it

seems to be getting worse. I fear that one day I might wake up and be unable to speak at all.

A: The core issue here is the fear and belief that stuttering could lead to mutism. This fear stems from something called autosuggestion (or self-hypnosis), which originates from your mind. An unsupervised and untrained mind can wield enough power to make you believe in nearly any illusion, even triggering seemingly inexplicable mental and physical conditions. Your personal reality and experiences aren't shaped solely by repetitive, scary thoughts but by the emotional investment you place in them – through anxiety and overthinking. This emotional charge turns these thoughts into a vivid anticipation of the very scenario you most fear. Ironically, the more we resist or reject an outcome, the more energy we pour into it, making it seem more likely to manifest.

Here's what I encourage you to do: intentionally choose your thoughts and focus your imagination on the life you want for yourself.

Imagine yourself living without this problem. How would you feel? How would you act and respond in various situations? What kind of thoughts would fill your mind in that state? Add rich detail to this visualization, making the experience as vivid and real as possible – like you're already living it. Make it a daily habit to actively focus on these positive, empowering thoughts while gently letting go of the ones you don't want.

Remember the formula I've shared before:

Think → Do (Experience) → Become.

Think the thoughts you want to cultivate now. Feel as though you're already the person you aspire to be. In doing so, you're mentally creating your desired experience, and over time you'll embody and become that version of yourself.

It's simple yet profound: thoughts of undesired scenarios lead to undesired outcomes. But the opposite is also true – thoughts of desired scenarios pave the way for the outcomes and experiences you truly wish to create.

Question 25:

Why your advice against complaining? I've been a lifelong PWS, and it helps to talk about it. Yes, sometimes I do complain, even with a positive mindset.

A: Complaining doesn't align with a positive mindset. People complain when they feel upset or burdened by problems, which is understandable – would anyone complain if there were nothing to complain about? Venting may offer temporary relief, but over time it often reinforces the problem, making it more entrenched and obscuring the way forward. Complaints can create a mental loop that prevents you from achieving lasting freedom and peace.

Once you begin to understand your stuttering – or any challenge, for that matter – and gain conscious control over it, complaining will lose its appeal. Instead, your energy will naturally shift towards taking exciting daily steps to restore your speech, build meaningful connections and uncover your truest self.

It's also important to acknowledge that, strangely, complaining about one's struggles can offer a subtle form of pleasure for many people, which is why they might continue to do it. But the process of recovery and growing out of speech anxiety is about making new choices – and choosing to step out of that cycle is one of them. Remember, not making a choice is still a choice.

'Once I realized that the world is indifferent to me and what I post on social media, I didn't feel despair. Instead, I felt a wave of relief wash over me. It was this liberating, air-punching moment when I finally understood – I can become anybody. I alone get to decide who I am and how I live. There's nothing standing in my way, only me – it's only ever been me.'

— Olga Bednarski

Question 26:

I'm currently taking an improv/acting basics class and am considering quitting, even though I love theatre and comedy. My stuttering, which fluctuates, worsened significantly at the start of this class, making it hard to perform. A year ago, I wouldn't have cared and would have pushed through. My current classmates are kind and haven't mentioned my stutter, but I worry that it might slow them down, even though they're very supportive. It feels unfair to them since they didn't sign up for a class with someone who stutters. Given these circumstances, what do you think is the right thing to do?

A: You're bullying yourself into leaving, believing that you're unworthy of being among these people. There's a clear and very evident pattern in what you described, and it goes like this. First, you try to convince yourself that 'I worry it might slow them down' and that it's 'unfair to them since they didn't sign up for a class with someone who stutters.' These are the narratives you've made up, and now you're trying to convince yourself of them. What happens next is in line with these worries, and it literally prevents you from being part of the theatre group that you enjoy. By doing this, you make yourself feel bad, guilty, defective and undeserving of staying (self-exclusion as punishment). This, in turn, unfortunately worsens your stutter, which further validates your original narrative and provides more evidence that you must leave. Leaving here acts as your own self-administered punishment – self-exclusion (sentencing yourself to exclusion).

Given the circumstances I've described, providing a detailed review of your situation, there are two options: continue terrorizing yourself and self-exclude while hanging your head in shame, or wake up, consciously change your narrative (the story you tell yourself), stay and continue enjoying what you love to do! I want to draw your attention to the fact that the people in your group, from your own words, are 'kind and haven't mentioned my stutter'. So, it's fair to say that you're the only one contributing to your misery and suffering here. There's no one else doing this, so you have the power to stop it! I'm not saying this to judge you, but to help you recognize this pattern and choose a different way of relating to yourself. This situation illustrates that if we don't accept ourselves, lack self-love and believe we're 'less than', no amount of external validation, kindness or acceptance will ever fill that void. First and foremost, you must learn to be kind to yourself.

What do I mean by choosing differently? Focus on your purpose for being in this group – I'm guessing it's because you love theatre and enjoy performing. So, focus on that, and let it guide you every time you go there. Instead of worrying about how you might be a hindrance or how others might perceive you, remember that everyone attends the class for themselves – not to impress you or the instructor, but for their own growth and joy. Go there and be there for you! Let that be your intention. Be compassionate and understanding towards yourself and forgive yourself for imperfections.

Coming from a place of acceptance and self-compassion, you no longer have to 'push through' but can instead start enjoying what you love and feel like a legitimate part of this group.

You have the choice to continue bullying yourself into leaving, or you can use this situation as an opportunity to transform your relationship with yourself and start enjoying this activity that's clearly dear to you. You create your own experience, so choose carefully what you think and what you allow yourself to create. I hope you've noticed this pattern and will be able to make a more informed and loving choice.

'Beliefs are psychoactive.'

— Olga Bednarski

Question 27:

Is stuttering caused by fear of speaking?

A: Stuttering is not the fear of speaking, but a deeply ingrained fear of being you and expressing yourself in the world in the way you truly want and are capable of.

It stems from a fear of invalidation, criticism, negative judgment and even physical punishment because, deep down, you carry an entrenched false belief that you're 'bad' and unworthy.

Essentially, this fear is the fear of your inner child, arising from a lack of parental love and acceptance. Because you don't feel fully accepted, loved or safe to be yourself, you hold back your voice, your expression and your creativity. As an adult, you end up seeking validation from others, hoping they'll tell you that 'you're okay', as you desperately try to be 'perfect' and 'worthy of love'. You continuously seek external approval, and the opinions of others seem more valid to you because you haven't yet fully learned to trust your own.

When you try to be perfect, you're not being real. Perfection becomes a mask, a shield, a straitjacket that hides your true self. Deep inside, you were led to believe that being authentic is unwelcome, embarrassing or even punishable. So instead, you present an edited, stunted version of yourself to the world, fully convinced that this is what must be accepted. But let me tell you, this could not be further from the truth.

Question 28:

How do you overcome fear and let yourself 'out of the cage' of perfection?

A: Learn to give yourself love. You do this by becoming your own ideal parent and friend – the parent who never criticizes, punishes or demands, but instead encourages and loves unconditionally. The friend who is always there to support, understand and embrace you, never to hold you back.

You must know, deep in your heart, that you'll always be there for yourself. No matter what. This is incredibly empowering!

As you learn to love yourself, your dependency on the support, praise, validation and attention of others gradually loosens. You'll feel safer to express yourself – both verbally and creatively. If you're a creative person, such as a musician or an artist, self-love is absolutely essential. Imagine how public criticism could silence you or make you feel invisible.

Self-love is one of the most powerful and meaningful goals in anyone's life. When you master the great skill of self-love, respect and acceptance, every area of your life will fall into a beautiful order and harmony.

Emotional regulation and anxiety management

Question 29:

Why do people interrupt me with 'what?' during my pauses when I'm speaking? It adds pressure and makes me feel misunderstood. I never do this to others when they're not finished speaking. Do people think I'm stupid?

A: It's not so much what people say, but how you choose to respond to it. If you feel added pressure, find yourself rushing to speak, losing your train of thought or feeling hurt, that's simply your current reaction. You may be reacting this way because you interpret their 'what?' as a sign of disrespect, invalidation or even an affront. In other words, you might be giving it too much significance and taking it personally. But here's the good news: you have the power to change how you perceive these moments and, in turn, how you feel, react and respond.

The first step is to attach a different meaning to their words. What if, instead of feeling pressured or misunderstood (or thinking they see you as 'stupid'), you choose to view it differently? Maybe they spaced out while you were speaking, got momentarily distracted or simply aren't great communicators themselves. What if, the next time you hear 'what?', you slow down on purpose, look them in the eyes, and say with a playful smile, '*Hello, are you even listening to me?*' By approaching it this way, you could lighten the moment, diffuse any tension and even laugh it off together.

While I don't know the full context of the situation from your question, it seems this isn't a formal or high-stakes environment – perhaps it's a casual meeting with friends or a conversation among teenagers. If that's the case, there's plenty of room for humour, and seriousness can take a back seat here. Let the next 'what?' you hear remind you to respond differently. Remember, your reaction is a choice. Use it as a gentle nudge to practise easing pressure rather than adding more.

Question 30:

I'm looking for tips to improve my performance in an online interview, where I'll be speaking in front of a group and answering questions with

other candidates. I've struggled in recent interviews, and I think my stammer is mainly due to anxiety, as I speak well when alone. Do you have any suggestions for reducing anxiety and speaking more confidently, especially in a competitive setting?

A: The pressure will ease, unlocking the natural flow you experience when speaking alone, once you stop viewing speech as a performance that must be perfect and stop taking it with such grave seriousness. Instead, approach it with a lighter attitude, focusing on connecting with people, interacting and conveying your message rather than trying to perform.

When your intention is to compete, impress or perform, the experience becomes emotionally and physically draining. You become overly attached to the outcome, placing unnecessary pressure on yourself, which leads to heightened anxiety. On the other hand, when your purpose shifts to connection and enjoyment, the outcome naturally becomes less significant. You let go of that attachment, mental strain eases, anxiety diminishes and your body loosens – no more rigidity or unnecessary muscular tension. Your breathing normalizes and, with it, your natural flow is freed.

To release this pressure and approach situations with greater ease, let go of the expectation of perfection. Before any interview or social event, forgive yourself in advance for however things might unfold. Embrace your humanness and imperfections and stop demanding perfection from yourself. Instead, focus on genuinely connecting with the people you meet. Trying to be perfect only creates an edited, stunted version of yourself, whereas authenticity fosters true connection.

Don't view this job opportunity as your last chance in the entire world. Avoid building it up with unrealistic hopes or expectations that you *must* get it, as though your existence depends on it. Letting go of such thoughts reduces pressure and allows you to remain grounded. Always have a Plan B so that you're not overly emotionally attached to the outcome of any interview or event. This shift in mindset will significantly reduce 'speech-performance-related' anxiety and boost your confidence.

In my programmes, I introduce the concept of play, which works wonders. Distract your mind from the pressure of speech and performance by stepping into playfulness. Turn the experience into a game. For example, as you speak, visualize what you're talking about in your mind's eye or imagine you're tasting chocolate as you speak, or walking on the beach. This playful approach instantly releases you from the performance trap and lets you be yourself. Play like a child – move towards presence, naturalness and peace. You can even play with pitch and tonality, treating your voice like a toy or an instrument.

Another way to make the situation more emotionally comfortable is to deliberately downplay its significance. See the people you're meeting not as intimidating figures there to judge you, but as fellow humans – friends even. Imagine the situation as a role play where you're playing the part of a job seeker in a grand charade or perhaps the main character on a talk show. Use this playful perspective to open up, flow naturally and stay present throughout the 'scene' so you can confidently present your skills and sell yourself to the employer.

And remember, even if you don't land this position, there are plenty of opportunities ahead. This isn't your last chance, not by any means. If things don't work out, don't beat yourself up. Treat it as another valuable learning experience that prepares you for the next time.

Lastly, verbal fluency alone doesn't guarantee a job. It's your authenticity that does the trick.

Question 31:

How do people who stutter overcome social anxiety and nervousness?

A: Social anxiety is, at its core, a fear of people that stems from an inability to accept and reconcile with yourself. It arises from the belief that you're not good enough and, therefore, have nothing valuable to offer in social situations. Genuine self-acceptance, however, begins with self-forgiveness and self-love. Without love and forgiveness, true acceptance can't exist.

Healing social anxiety requires learning to be compassionate, loving and unconditionally accepting towards yourself. Compassion isn't just a fleeting feeling – it's an attitude, as are acceptance and love. Unlike emotions, which ebb and flow, attitudes can be cultivated, invited and nurtured, even in the face of challenging emotional states or external events. When you approach yourself with compassion and love, there's no room for harsh self-judgment or the pressure to conform to societal standards in order to feel worthy. You begin to see and accept yourself fully, exactly as you are. And, in turn, you find it easier to accept others in the same way.

Through compassion and unconditional love, whatever emotions or thoughts arise within you can be met with curiosity rather than frustration or impatience. This shift allows you to engage in what I call a 'reality check'. A reality check helps you step back and objectively evaluate the validity of your thoughts and perceptions. Often, you'll discover that many of these mental constructions are subjective and context-bound – they feel real within a specific frame of mind but lack universal truth. With this realization, you gain the freedom to disentangle yourself from these constructs, no longer bound by their limitations.

When you learn to love yourself, to consistently be on your own side no matter the external circumstances, your entire state of being transforms. You stand taller, both metaphorically and literally, as your confidence grows. Social anxiety and irrational nervousness – once overwhelming – begin to diminish and eventually fade away entirely.

Love truly creates magic in your life. It heals not just social anxiety or speech anxiety, but all aspects of your experience. That's why it's so vital to devote your energy to understanding and mastering the powerful art of self-love.

My own social anxiety disorder disappeared when I finally stopped imposing impossible standards of perfection on myself. I let go of the exhausting habit of trying to anticipate what others expected of me and striving to meet those imagined demands. Instead, I gave myself permission to simply be me. I stopped criticising myself and let myself exist in peace. This shift in perception brought about a profound transformation. It resolved many challenges in my life, filling me with an enduring sense of presence and inner peace. The heavy burden of conditionality I had carried for years was lifted, leaving me free to breathe, to grow and to align with myself – mentally, emotionally and spiritually.

Love is the essential fifth element we so often overlook – the element of creation itself. Without it, nothing could exist.

'Liberation is really nothing but the personality becoming free in the moment; the personality loses its grip and allows itself to simply relax.'

— A.H. Almaas

Question 32:

I've been speaking much better than usual for months, but now I'm struggling to get words out. I don't understand why this is happening.

A: As I mentioned earlier, it's worth reflecting on the times when your speech flowed more smoothly, paying close attention to your emotional and physical states during those periods. The better you feel, the better you speak. Stuttering is a mind-driven pattern, often sustained by repetitive thoughts. Therefore, I believe that during times of improved speech, your mind is naturally distracted from habitual ruminations about speaking and redirected towards more engaging and fulfilling activities or events.

Ruminations – usually tinged with anxiety – disrupt your inner emotional balance and, in turn, affect the natural rhythm of your speech. By carefully observing yourself during moments of ease compared to times of difficulty, you can start to identify what drives these shifts. As your self-awareness grows, you'll become better equipped to maintain inner balance and sustain your flow.

Here are some key areas to focus on in your self-observation:

- **Inner Self-Talk:** Pay attention to the dialogue running through your mind, especially before entering situations where you anticipate speaking. How are you framing the situation? Are you predicting success or fearing failure?
- **Breathing Patterns:** Notice whether your breathing is shallow and erratic, as this can disrupt speech flow. Establish a natural, deep and full breathing pattern, not only before speaking but throughout the day. Full, steady breaths set the foundation for calm and flowing communication.
- **Attention and Focus:** Often, PWS, like most habitual worriers, tend to live in their heads – overthinking, ruminating and anticipating negative outcomes. Shift your focus to the present moment. You can do this by observing your breath, noticing the sensation of fabric on your skin, tasting the food in your mouth or simply taking in the colours, shapes and textures of your surroundings. Avoid judging or interpreting; just observe. A simple question like, 'Am I present, or am I caught up in unconscious thoughts?' can be incredibly grounding. The moment you realize you're not present, you are. Allow yourself to simply be.
- **Reactions to Events and People:** Take note of how certain situations or individuals make you feel. If specific reactions cause you to shrink inwardly or wish to avoid the moment, explore the thoughts and beliefs fuelling these responses. Consider how you might reframe or change your perspective on them.

These practices should become part of your daily self-awareness routine. Developing an understanding of what influences your inner state and speech patterns will help you uncover the reasons for fluctuations in your speech. From there, you can learn to adjust – for example, returning to deep, even breathing, slowing your pace, pausing before speaking or replacing negative self-talk with affirming, supportive thoughts.

The tools and practices I suggest are designed to train your mind, so it becomes a powerful tool you can use, rather than letting your mind control you.

Remember, the effectiveness of these practices lies in consistent and committed application.

Question 33:

Has anyone found that their speech has improved over the years but that they experience more anxiety because of this improvement? How do you manage this anxiety and fear of failure?

A: Here's a simple mental trick. To minimize and avoid provoking anxiety (fear) of losing your fluency, I encourage you not to become overly ecstatic or euphoric when it arrives. Similarly, try not to feel too disheartened or devastated when turbulence arises. Strong emotional fluctuations – whether positive or negative – can unintentionally feed the problem. Instead, aim to remain calm and as neutral as possible.

To expand further on this, here's what I would like to share. It's most likely the fear of losing what you've gained – your fluency. And, if I were to guess, this fear might be tied to a deeper worry: falling from grace, leading to what feels like social demise. You might fear being seen as a failure or disappointing those who have supported you, those who hoped you were permanently 'cured'.

But here's the truth: when you become consciously aware of how your speech anxiety operates – when you understand your triggers and develop the ability to self-regulate – you'll no longer experience this fear of loss. There will be no reason to fear because you'll know how to course-correct and stabilize yourself during times of turbulence. And, over time, those turbulent moments will become less frequent and far less daunting.

Your fluency – your natural flow – cannot be lost. That belief itself is a limiting idea. Fluency has always been with you, waiting patiently beneath layers of mental clutter: false beliefs, disempowering stories you've told yourself (or absorbed from others over the years) and the endless noise of misinformation that perpetuates the myth that stuttering is some exotic, incurable condition.

When you stop being mesmerized by the collective unconsciousness – when you awaken from the trance of popular opinions and rigid scientific theories – you'll see the truth clearly. You'll understand, in practice, how you've been creating the experience of anxiety and stuttering.

And once you become conscious of that, there will be nothing left to fear.

Question 34:

How can I keep myself calm? Could you suggest any effective strategies for managing nerves?

A: Consciously choose what to think, and create future memories as if your desired outcomes – such as your confidence and fluency – are already here with you. Think and feel as though you're the person who already possesses everything you want. Keep imagining the desired scenario in your mind, adding more details to make it feel real. Fuel it with your active imagination and visualization – this is the same process you use to create negative scenarios and anxiety.

Anticipate success, rehearse positivity, and not failure. This is a skill, and like any skill it requires practice to develop. Don't be disheartened if it doesn't work the first time. With consistent effort, you'll learn to self-regulate and tune into this mindset at will. This practice taps into the power of neuroplasticity.

For further details and ideas, feel free to read and re-read my responses to other questions.

Question 35:

How do you deal with the shame of stuttering?

A: Stop feeling ashamed and start being on your own side. Always offer yourself support and compassion. Learn from the mistakes you've made, apologize to those you've hurt, but never gaslight or bully yourself. Be your own ally. This mindset should become your lifestyle.

PWS often become masters at torturing themselves on demand, but the practice of being on your own side will reverse this and teach you self-love. This skill is fundamental in dissolving any kind of anxiety, not just speech anxiety.

'You become more you as you let go of everything that isn't truly you.'

— Olga Bednarski, author of *The Anatomy of Stuttering*

Question 36:

I love that I never stutter when I'm angry. I can't say my name when asked, but if someone makes me angry enough, I unleash my fury with 100 per cent fluency. How does it happen?

A: That's the healing power of letting go. When what you truly want to say – your message – takes centre stage in your mind, stuttering is pushed aside. You stop holding back, and the trigger, that tight feeling in your gut, is released. In that moment, you're 'healed' from stuttering, and speech flows naturally. On a mental level, you disidentify from stuttering and the usual behaviours that this self-identification forces you to follow. You become free.

I hear about such 'healings' all the time. This example beautifully illustrates how stuttering (holding back) is merely a rigid mental construct, a learned habit or even an illusion. Instead of being fleeting, these healings can be sustained, as long as you understand how stuttering works (see *The Anatomy of Stuttering*) and learn to self-regulate your emotions.

As a mental construct or learned behaviour, the degree to which people identify with it varies. The more you can detach from identifying with your stuttering, the sooner you'll replace the behaviours that keep it in place – and ultimately eliminate it from your life.

Social interactions and relationships

Question 37:

As a nervous and sensitive person, I'm a true empath and introvert. What bothers me most is not meeting strangers but having conversations with loved ones where I stutter more, fear being interrupted and then get cut off. My elderly mother, despite being a speech and language pathologist, still interrupts me and changes the subject mid-sentence. I'm turning 65 in August, and being her care-giver is stressful enough without these interruptions. Can I at least finish my thoughts?

A: You do not receive what you deserve – you accept what you're willing to put up with. This applies to all relationships, including those with family. I believe the situation you're describing, where you feel dismissed, likely has its roots in your childhood and didn't just start recently. It's fair to say your mother may have always been authoritative and perhaps overbearing, regardless of her education. I have known some highly qualified teachers whose treatment of their own children was, frankly, abysmal.

When a mother is overbearing, dismissive or emotionally volatile, a child often adapts by shrinking into near invisibility – becoming quiet and unobtrusive to avoid trouble or, worse, punishment. Growing up in such an environment can make children hypersensitive and constantly on edge, nervously anticipating a parental mood swing or outburst. Because children tend to internalize blame, they assume their parent's unhappiness is their fault. They do whatever they can to avoid provoking anger, striving to remain quiet, compliant and invisible in hopes of staying loved, accepted and safe.

I suspect that as a child you weren't truly listened to and that your opinions were often dismissed. This would have been deeply traumatic for a child, as we're innately wired for connection and attachment. Being ignored or invalidated in this way would have left emotional scars that still linger today.

It's clear that your mother – and perhaps other close family members – weren't, and still aren't, the sources of support, attention and understanding you needed. There may have been times when you sought help or compassion, only to be met with indifference, harsh reprimands or even rejection. Such experiences send a painful message to a child: '*You don't matter. Your feelings and needs aren't important.*'

Over time, you likely learned to suppress your emotions entirely, becoming accommodating and putting up with whatever treatment came your way. This pattern, learned in childhood, became deeply ingrained, and even now, when you approach loved ones, you may find yourself freezing, stalling or withdrawing – feeling like that same dismissed little boy or girl. It's as though you're being transported back in time. Unfortunately, emotional memories don't come with expiration dates, so they continue to affect you, regardless of your age.

This behavioural and emotional adaptation often carries into adulthood, leaving you feeling stuck – accommodating, quiet, invisible and yet deeply unhappy. Even as an adult, the automatic anticipation of being interrupted, dismissed or ignored can trigger anxiety and nervousness, especially when dealing with family members like your mother.

As I've mentioned before, suppressing your emotions stalls emotional growth. When we suppress our feelings, we remain stuck in the past, unable to mature and expand emotionally. It's no wonder you still feel like that guilty little child around your mother, powerless and unable to change anything. People who habitually suppress their needs often accumulate not just anxiety but also anger or even rage. As you can imagine, there's no room for self-love in this cycle.

But here's the key: you *can* choose how to respond now, because you're an adult. If not now, when? After all, you're already 63. Don't expect your mother – or anyone else – to suddenly change and acknowledge your needs. She hasn't done it before, and she won't start now. If you're holding on to the hope that she might one day become the understanding and patient listener you've always wanted, let go of that expectation. It will only keep you stuck.

To change this dynamic, you need to adjust your approach and take responsibility for your own growth.

My advice? Don't waste any more time hoping your mother will change. Instead, focus on changing how you respond. When she interrupts, dismiss her interruptions as though you didn't hear them. Keep speaking and finish your sentence. It's important to give yourself permission to speak and stand firm in your right to be heard.

It feels to me like you still interpret her interruptions as signals to stop talking – just as you did in childhood. But recognize that you are a fully fledged adult now. Don't let those old, learned behaviours hold you back. Speak with confidence, self-respect and assertion. Nobody can take away your right to speak – only you can do that by staying silent.

As another piece of advice to consider: Have you shown yourself empathy for all you've endured? Have you tried sharing responsibility for her care with others, such as siblings or extended family, if that's an option? You deserve support, not just from others but also from yourself.

Ultimately, the choice is yours. If you don't change your attitude or take steps to introduce these changes, nothing will change. You don't receive what you deserve – you receive what you accept.

Question 38:

I've been told that I'm a good person to talk to, as my friends often come to me during tough times. Is being able to understand what it's like to hurt and be judged a strength?

A: It's a wonderful strength to be empathetic and eager to help others. However, if you forget about yourself, constantly sacrificing your own needs and plans to answer every call for help, this strength can turn into a festering issue. Over time, it may leave you feeling used, resentful and overwhelmed with anger or frustration.

Let me explain. It all comes down to self-love. Ask yourself: am I helping out of love, or for love?

A lack of self-love – self-respect, self-appreciation – is one of the most common challenges for PWS. Often, this leads to a reliance on external validation. You might find yourself depending heavily on others to approve of you, to praise you, to accept you or to make you feel like you're 'good enough'. Sometimes, this need even stems from avoiding feelings of guilt. This pattern often develops subconsciously, shaped by how we were treated as children.

If our parents or caregivers were loving, supportive and took us seriously as children, we grow up with a solid foundation of self-worth. We develop internal roots, like a tree. When those roots are strong, we're resilient and self-reliant. We don't feel the need to seek constant approval or validation from others. But if those roots weren't nurtured, we often look for validation outside ourselves, playing what I call the 'niceness game'. This game can be exhausting and comes at the cost of our own well-being, plans and desires.

Don't get me wrong – there's nothing wrong with wanting to help others. Listening, supporting and being there in moments of crisis is a beautiful thing. But here's the key: you must be able to discern why you're helping. Are you doing it purely from the kindness of your heart, because you truly want to? Or are you doing it to gain praise, gratitude or validation?

If your help comes from genuine kindness and love, then it's healthy and fulfilling – for both you and the person you're helping. But if you find yourself feeling resentful or hurt when someone doesn't show you the appreciation you expected, it's worth reflecting. In that case, you may have helped for love, hoping for emotional 'payment' in return. This type of giving can be draining, creating feelings of bitterness over time.

There will always be moments when loved ones need urgent help, and of course it's natural to occasionally set aside your plans to be there for them. But here's an important question to ask yourself: if I refused to help for a valid reason, would I feel guilty?

If the answer is yes, then that guilt is a warning sign. Constantly sacrificing your own needs to help others will eventually leave you feeling depleted and taken for granted. This isn't a healthy or sustainable way to give. You need to tend to your own needs and honour your own plans first.

To ensure your help is both meaningful and balanced, these three conditions should always be met:

1. They ask for your help (don't help if nobody asked you)
2. You want to help.
3. You can help.

If these three conditions aren't in place, consider stepping back. Don't impose your help if it hasn't been requested, and don't feel pressured to sacrifice yourself. True kindness doesn't come with strings attached. You're not responsible for everyone's happiness, nor should you feel obligated to fix every problem.

For PWS, empathy can be a remarkable strength when used wisely. But without healthy boundaries it can become a weakness, leaving you feeling like a doormat – or worse, an emotional dumping ground. Protect your energy by setting those boundaries. Help because you want to, and because you can.

If someone ever tries to manipulate you with ultimatums – for example, by saying they won't be your friend unless you listen to them or help them – you must decide whether that's the kind of friendship you truly want. Genuine friends don't use or manipulate you.

Above all, remember this: help out of love, not for love.

'Go from blaming to cherishing, from hatred to love and acceptance.'

— Olga Bednarski

Question 39:

I often blame my strong personality and feel stuck in a cycle. I tell myself to speak less, but as a social person I struggle to hold back. While I start relationships well, I quickly worry that people dislike me. When I need to speak up, I sometimes stay silent to avoid discomfort. Why do I keep doing this, especially when even my family struggles to understand me?

A: The answer to your turmoil lies within your question. You're trying to force yourself into being someone you're not, squeezing yourself into a straitjacket to meet some perceived societal standards and expectations. The harder you push, the more you suffer – anxiety, depression and inner turmoil – because you're standing in the way of your own greatness and authenticity. Do you really want to keep restricting yourself, confining your spirit within the tight constraints of these self-imposed boundaries? Is this prison of self-rejection the life you wish to live?

To break free and end this cycle of suffering, you must begin by accepting yourself. Become your own best friend, someone who loves and supports you unconditionally. Let yourself be. Stop suppressing the powerful, fiery lion within you. If you keep trying to push that fire down, you risk burning yourself out from the inside, destroying your happiness and dimming your light.

Picture yourself as a mighty oak tree. Now imagine if that oak began clipping its own branches day by day, trying to shrink itself to fit in with the smaller, weaker trees and bushes around it. Over time, what would be left of the majestic oak? It would lose its grandeur and might not even resemble a tree anymore.

That is what you're doing to yourself when you try to fit in by rejecting or hiding who you truly are. If you reject yourself, don't be surprised if others do the same – they're simply reflecting your own relationship with yourself. When you feel disliked or rejected, remember that the world often mirrors how you treat yourself.

For many, stuttering stems from holding back – repressing emotions, words or truths. To overcome it, you must do the opposite: stop clipping your own wings to blend in and instead spread them wide. Accept and embrace yourself as you are. Set the intention to be your own best friend – the kind of friend who is always on your side, who listens, supports, forgives and understands no matter what.

When I overcame my anxiety, I realized that during all those years of trying to fit in, to earn external love and acceptance, I was diminishing myself. I was cutting away parts of who I truly was, suppressing my greatest strengths and unique qualities. I believed these traits were flaws to be hidden, but they turned out to be my most valuable assets. They were the keys to unlocking opportunities and fulfilment in my life. I was stealing from myself, disowning parts of my being, which only deepened the disconnection I felt – a spiritual void that no external validation could ever fill.

Inside me was a nuclear power, a force waiting to be unleashed. Suppressing it only made me feel like I was on the verge of exploding. Peace only came when I embraced it.

You can't reject or suppress the power within you – it's unstoppable. The only way forward is to embrace it and let it guide you. You'll only find true love when you learn to love yourself. You'll only feel truly accepted when you accept yourself. You're an angel – why insist on living the life of a duck? Why stoop low like a bush when you can stand tall as the mighty oak that you already are?

The root of the problem lies in your mind, in self-rejection and the inability to accept yourself. From there, it spreads into every area of your life, stealing your inner peace, dulling your joy and complicating your relationships with others. But the solution also begins in your mind: choosing to accept, understand and cherish yourself.

Question 40:

My relationship ended because of my stuttering, which I always feared. Has anyone else experienced this? How did you handle it?

A: Anticipating a problem often leads to its manifestation. Be mindful of what you focus on, because once it becomes your reality, it's hard to complain – you invited it in.

This is a classic example of a self-fulfilling prophecy, where you attract what you fear most. The more you dwell on the events that make you anxious, the more likely they are to show up in your life. This is the law of resonance at work. It's not just about thoughts – your negative feelings and vivid mental images of worst-case scenarios create a powerful energy that aligns with unpleasant outcomes, drawing them closer to you.

To change this pattern, take some time to sit with yourself and reflect honestly. Ask yourself: Why do I believe I don't deserve to be loved? Why do I see myself as unlovable or unlucky in relationships? Why do I anticipate people leaving me? And most importantly, what does this say about my relationship with myself?

Life and the people around us are mirrors – they reflect back what we carry inside: our beliefs, attitudes and self-perceptions. Everything starts with you and ends with you.

As for your stuttering, I don't believe it's the root cause of the challenges you're experiencing. Instead, it's likely how much weight you give it. If it takes centre stage in your relationships – where you're constantly worrying about your speech and agonizing over it – it can be difficult to show up as your authentic self. When your speech becomes the focus, it can overshadow everything else, making it challenging for others to see the amazing person you truly are.

Rather than fearing people will leave you, imagine the opposite. Picture people being drawn to you, enjoying your company and wanting to be around you. Visualize these moments vividly – feel the joy, warmth and connection of those scenarios. By consciously choosing positive thoughts and feelings, you create a new energy that can attract more uplifting experiences into your life.

Look around you: there are so many people with visible disabilities, and they find love and deep connections. Stuttering isn't as significant a barrier as you might think – unless you give it that power. It's all about perspective.

I don't know your exact age, but I imagine you're very young. My advice? Don't let speech anxiety take the lead role in your life.

Question 41:

I don't have any friends in real life because of my stuttering. What to do?

A: If you know at least one person who stutters and has friends, then your lack of friends has nothing to do with your stuttering. It stems more from your beliefs and the actions – or inactions – that arise from those beliefs and an erroneous self-perception.

What steps are you taking to build real-life friendships? Do you go out and engage with others? Where can people meet you? Holding on to the idea that your life will improve without your active participation is a recipe for stagnation. I hate to break it to you, but it doesn't work that way. Change and improvement happen when you open yourself up to life and take small, courageous steps towards the life you want. Even the smallest steps matter. And when you take one step towards life, life often takes ten steps towards you.

You don't have to remain home alone; you can find your community. But it requires action – a commitment to change and the courage to show up. Muster your bravery and take yourself to a social event. It might feel daunting at first, but I promise it gets easier after the initial try. If you hide from life, life hides from you.

There are many platforms to help you connect with others. For example, Meetup.com offers countless social events in cities around the world. These events are wonderful opportunities to experiment, step outside your comfort zone and hone your social skills. Nobody knows you there, which means you have the freedom to be whoever you want to be. Don't let stuttering or anxiety rob you of the joy of interacting with others and building meaningful connections.

I understand stepping out of your comfort zone can feel intimidating, but ask yourself: would you rather endure the pain of loneliness or face the temporary discomfort of showing up for life? Don't let yourself fall into self-induced suffering and isolation, which is a trap many PWS unknowingly set for themselves. Grant yourself permission to enjoy friendships and the pleasure of social interactions.

You can support yourself by speaking uplifting words to yourself – this is called intentional thinking. Forgive yourself in advance for any imperfections, embracing your humanity and vulnerability. This will make it easier, psychologically and emotionally, to come out of your shell and show up in the world.

Your mind has created the story of your loneliness. You can use that same mind to intentionally craft a new story – one of sociability, attractiveness and, yes, even confidence in romantic pursuits, if that's what you desire.

Those who seek will always find.

Question 42:

How do you improve communication skills and interact normally? I've been shy and awkward my whole life, often stuttering so much I could barely breathe. Now, as an adult, I'm trying to speak and interact more but still struggle. How can I overcome this, especially given that my lack of social interaction during my teens due to my stutter affects me now?

A: Speech anxiety and the social awkwardness (or shyness) that often accompanies it can only be addressed by immersing yourself in social situations – facing what you fear. Social skills, like any other skill, can be learned and refined. But to truly grow and internalize these skills, you must adopt a hands-on approach and practise consistently. At first, this may feel uncomfortable or even artificial, but that discomfort will gradually fade when you do three important things: give yourself permission to be imperfect, stop seeing others merely as 'judges of your speech' and adopt a playful (or 'not give a shit') attitude towards social situations.

To ease perfectionism, start by granting yourself the permission to make mistakes. Learning any new skill involves trial and error – no one becomes an expert on their first try. Be patient and persistent, ready to experiment and try again. Your view of others will also shift when you consciously choose to seek support in people, rather than searching for signs of disapproval – be it in a disapproving look, a giggle or a raised eyebrow. Focus on finding allies and ignore anything that doesn't serve your growth. Lastly, approach social situations with a sense of playfulness rather than grave seriousness. The latter only increases tension and exacerbates feelings of awkwardness or insecurity. A playful attitude, on the other hand, dissolves stress, fosters openness and allows you to relax into being your authentic self. This shift naturally leads to smoother interactions, greater ease and more enjoyment.

Many PWS report feeling they lack finesse in social interactions – a sentiment I can deeply relate to. But it's important to recognize that there's no one-size-fits-all way to communicate effectively. Interaction styles are as unique as individuals. Some people are wonderfully eccentric and yet are embraced as fantastic communicators. This shows that authenticity, not conformity, is key.

To minimize discomfort, try replacing the habit of 'preparing for impact' with intentionally looking forward to social situations. Cultivate a sense of pleasant anticipation, anticipating positive outcomes instead of replaying past social challenges and projecting them into your future. At the heart of successful communication lies self-acceptance. And the foundation of genuine self-acceptance is self-love. The more you love yourself (which is very different from vanity or selfishness), the easier it becomes to connect with others. Self-love is a powerful, often-overlooked antidote.

Self-love is a mindset anyone can cultivate. All it requires is your intention and willingness to weave it into your daily life. By nurturing self-love, you transform your relationship with yourself, creating a new state of being. With consistent practice, even over a short period (two to three months), you'll witness remarkable changes – in your thoughts, your emotions, your experiences, and especially your social interactions.

Question 43:

I recently ended my relationship due to insecurity about my stuttering. He seemed okay with it, but I felt he didn't truly understand what I was going through. I don't want to repeat this pattern in future relationships. How can I address this issue?

A: You should start by deciding why you want to enter a relationship in the first place. Are you looking for a partner who will support you and be by your side? Or do you want to constantly educate your partner about stuttering, testing their understanding, seeking their constant support and watching out for signs of misunderstanding and lack of support? My advice would be to set your priorities straight. What do you want from relationships?

In your case, it seems that you may want your partner to engage more with your stuttering than with you as a person. This indicates an emotional immaturity I spoke about earlier, and self-centredness. Stuttering should take a back seat in your relationship for it to work. It seems like you've confused your identity with your stuttering. Don't you think? This is an example of how people, over time, can unknowingly become so fully identified with their problems that they 'become' their problem. This isn't limited to stuttering – it can apply to any challenge we face.

Imagine how it must feel for your partner, constantly being suspected of lacking understanding or being asked for empathy. Have you ever considered their feelings? Would you want to be in a relationship with someone whose primary focus is their own struggle, where their insecurities take centre stage and they complain and create drama about it, maybe even daily? Probably not. If you don't want to deal with your partner's insecurities, it's important to first address your own.

If you want to have joyful and fulfilling relationships with others, you should cultivate a different relationship with yourself. Downgrade your impediment from its current VIP status in your life. Otherwise, you risk having a relationship with your stuttering alone. Choose better for yourself.

We live in the world we imagine for ourselves. Choose what you want to imagine.

And if you don't want to repeat this pattern, you don't have to.

Question 44:

I was shamed and reprimanded while speaking with stutter, is that why I developer stuttering?

A: There's more to it than that. Your whole being – your very self – was subjected to scrutiny, judgment and perhaps even physical punishment. As a result of these experiences, a child may come to an unfortunate conclusion: 'I'm not good enough, I'm bad.'

This belief leads the child to begin to 'shrink', suppressing their personality, emotions and speech. Speaking is a tool for self-expression, a way to be heard in the world. If you believe you're not good enough, would you speak up? Of course not.

Instead, you would suppress your voice and shrink into the background, hoping to become invisible so you can avoid judgment and be 'good'. Stuttering is the result of all that suppression. Sadly, only a rare parent understands the intricacies of a child's emotional development.

In my own teens, in addition to stuttering, I developed a skin-picking disorder. I picked at my facial skin until it was raw and damaged. I believed I was so bad and unworthy that I had no right to exist. I pressed and suppressed myself in every way I could imagine. All of these were coping strategies, attempts to shield myself from feelings I didn't know how to handle. Anxiety came first, and all the coping mechanisms followed.

Question 45:

How can I cope with the difficulty and pain of talking to my family, who I feel don't understand my suffering and tend to be judgemental, especially when I stutter in front of them. How can I address my feelings of being unfairly compared to my siblings and my hope that moving away might help me overcome my stutter?

A: What can truly help alleviate your suffering in this situation is to release the expectation that they'll understand you.

If they haven't understood you before, they're unlikely to understand you now or in the future. Holding on to the hope for their understanding and support keeps you emotionally tethered and contributes to your daily suffering. You might not even realize it, but their understanding has become a condition for your happiness. It's as if you're telling yourself, 'Unless my family understands me, I can't be happy or at peace with myself.'

Let go of this condition – the ball and chain tied to your leg that drags you down. Intend to accept yourself as you are, independent of their understanding or support. Choose to be your own source of understanding, kindness and encouragement. Always be on your side.

We've been taught to believe that without the acceptance of others, even from our family, we somehow lack the right to accept ourselves, to embrace who we are and even to live fully. But the truth is the opposite: before anyone else can truly accept you, you must first accept, understand and love yourself.

This shift in perspective will bring immediate relief, emotional independence and, over time, freedom. If you see yourself as the 'odd one out' or the 'black sheep' in your family, you may come to discover that this is actually a hidden blessing – one that reveals itself once you embrace and accept yourself fully.

Moving away from your family might indeed be a step towards independence and personal growth. However, don't do it as a means to overcome stuttering; do it for you – for your growth, your development and your advancement as a person.

Now is the time for action. The journey begins with you!

Question 46:

How can I overcome the anxiety of speaking with people in authority or speaking in front of a crowd?

A: Give yourself permission to be whoever you want to be or whoever you feel you truly are. Balance their authority with your own. Feel the strength of your own authority. Now step into the situation as an equal – no matter who they are – without diminishing yourself or feeling smaller. Notice how this shift in mindset can profoundly transform your experience.

The same applies to public speaking: empower yourself to take the stage and confidently deliver your message. Trust in your right to be there and let your voice be heard.

Question 47:

Why is speaking to my parents and close ones so much harder for me, with frequent blocks, compared to speaking to stranger. How can I overcome this issue?

A: Give yourself permission to be whoever you want to be or whoever you feel you truly are. Balance their authority with your own. Feel the strength of your own authority. Now step into the situation as an equal – no matter who they are – without diminishing yourself or feeling smaller. Notice how this shift in mindset can profoundly transform your experience.

The same applies to public speaking: empower yourself to take the stage and confidently deliver your message. Trust in your right to be there and let your voice be heard.

Question 48:

Why do I find it so hard to speak to my mother, with increased speech blocks and being unable to utter a sound? Will I always be 'Mummy's stuttering boy', and how can I decrease my stuttering in these situations?

A: You find it difficult to speak with your mother because, each time you do, you're emotionally transported back to the role of a little 'Mummy's stuttering boy'. It's not the adult you who stands before her; it's that inner child who still feels small and unsure. If your mother has been emotionally cold, volatile or critical, imagine how that inner child reacts – feeling scared, shrinking, suppressing emotions and growing anxious. This shift in your emotional state immediately affects your ability to express yourself, including your speech.

This experience is deeply subjective because it's rooted in emotion, not logic. So, if you want to better understand it and reduce your anxiety when speaking with your mother, step away from rationalizing. Instead, focus on the feelings that arise and how they influence your responses.

Without realizing it, you may still play the role of the well-behaved boy trying to please his mother. In doing so, you're not being your authentic self, which creates mental and physical tension and exacerbates your stuttering. This behaviour likely stems from a deep desire to maintain attachment to her – an attachment that was crucial for your survival as a child but is no longer necessary now that you're an adult.

Your stuttering, or holding back, can lessen when you consciously step into your role as the adult you are today. Recognize that you]re no longer helpless or dependent on your mother for survival (I hope so). Let go of any expectation that she'll change or suddenly provide what she couldn't give you as a child – whether that's love, appreciation or understanding. Release the tendency to idolize her; nobody is perfect, and that's okay.

Choose to grow beyond the role of the little boy and begin embodying the adult you've become. Ask yourself: How would the adult version of me relate to my relationship with my mother? What would his feelings, emotions, attitudes and responses be? Write it all down to bring clarity to your thoughts.

This transition may feel emotionally risky at first, so take it step by step.

Self-love and acceptance

Question 49:

How can I relieve the pressure to speak properly, which has recently made me stutter on almost every letter, even though I accept and am content with my stuttering?

A: Most, if not all, PWS fall into a common trap – trying not to stutter. In doing so, they overfocus and overthink their speech, triggering a cycle that inevitably leads to more struggle, more blocking and sometimes even a complete inability to utter a word – a silent block. This mental overpreparation for speaking primes your entire system – your mind, your breathing patterns and your body – for stuttering.

What we focus on expands. The more you think about, resist or resent something undesirable, the more it manifests in your experience. If you don't catch yourself in time and break the cycle, it can consume your mental space and even your life, turning into a manic obsession. This principle doesn't apply only to speaking; it's universal and can influence every area of life.

If you truly accept and feel at peace with your stuttering, why would you pressure yourself to 'speak properly'? Why place such heavy expectations on yourself? Speak as your speech wants to come out. Simply allow the sounds to flow in their own way, without judgment or an imagined need to meet the expectations of others.

It's the extra, self-inflicted pressure that causes most of the difficulties for PWS – pressure that can often be avoided by simply letting go. Let the process of speaking unfold naturally, however it will. The key is recognizing how you might unintentionally get in your own way and then making a conscious decision to stop doing so.

This isn't always easy at first, but by reading these words and acknowledging this tendency, you're already halfway there. To step aside and allow your speech to flow, you'll need to learn to negotiate with yourself. This might feel like coaxing a small child, gently reassuring your mind. Remind yourself that your body already knows how to produce sounds and words. There's no need to place expectations on yourself to speak in any special way other than what feels natural – whether that includes stumbles, long pauses or even moments of silence.

Forgive yourself in advance for any stumbles or mishaps that may arise in speaking situations. Sincere self-forgiveness can lift a tremendous weight off your shoulders and remove much of the pressure and easy perfectionism. With that weight gone, you can move forward with greater ease.

It's important to note that developing these self-negotiation (or self-coaching) skills – essentially quieting your inner 'monkey mind' – takes time and practice. But with consistent effort, it won't take long. Many skilled speakers and negotiators use this technique, which helps them remain composed and 'unmoved' even during heated debates. Once learned, this skill becomes a lifelong asset.

Question 50:

As a child struggling with my stutter, I often wondered, Why me? What did I do to deserve this? Over the years, I've found some comfort in understanding that it's a neurological condition, likely genetic from my maternal side since two of my mum's four brothers also stuttered. I've come to terms with it and try to stay positive, even if I feel awkward when stuttering with strangers.

I've recently experienced sleep deprivation from staying up late and compensating with strong coffee. I've noticed that these changes seem to increase my speech hesitation and blocking. Is this a common experience, and are there any strategies to manage it?

A: First of all, I can sense a bit of inner conflict in how you're relating to your stuttering. On one hand, you've found comfort in thinking it's a genetic condition (which, by the way, it's not), and on the other hand, you feel awkward when stuttering with strangers. There's either acceptance or unacceptance – there's no middle ground.

Deceiving yourself is one of the hardest things to do. Once you fully accept your challenge, you won't feel awkward or uncomfortable showing it. Take, for example, Nick Vujicic, a man born with the rare condition tetra-Amelia syndrome, which means he was born without arms or legs. Despite initially struggling with his condition, even attempting to drown himself in the bathtub, he eventually accepted and embraced his reality. Once he stopped agonizing over his limitations and stopped wishing them away, he began to see the opportunities in his life. He focused on what he could offer the world instead of what he lacked. His passion for life and sense of humour are truly inspiring. He went on to become a motivational speaker and a living testament to the incredible power of the human spirit. You might think it's a miracle – but it's not. It's what we can achieve when we stop letting our problems steal our precious energy, time and meaning. That is our life.

To me, this is about what you prioritize. You can choose to focus on your problem while being a perfectly able-bodied person, or you can choose to stop suffering and hating yourself for it. If you choose to prioritize your happiness and lead a fulfilling life, you'll find a way to get there – by choice, with determination and with acceptance. Alternatively, if you decide to make your life difficult, that will be your reality.

I mentioned this at the start of the book, and I don't want to dwell on it too much here, but just as a reminder: the only 'genetic' aspect of stuttering is the temperament we inherit from our parents. Our genes are activated by the environment and its impact on us. People who develop speech anxiety tend to be naturally more sensitive, which makes them more acutely affected by environmental influences. This explains the stuttering in your mother's two brothers as well.

Given your own heightened sensitivity, along with similar environmental factors in your upbringing, it's not surprising that stuttering developed for you, too. The experiences you had growing up, the quality of your relationships with your parents and the environmental triggers all played a role.

Sleep deprivation and speech hesitation

Some people report that sleep deprivation improves their speech, while others say it contributes to more blocking. In your case, here's what I want to say: sleep deprivation leads to tiredness, which invites you to slow down and relax, urging you to rest and recharge your energy. Tiredness physically softens you, loosens you up and calms your nervous system in preparation for rest.

For someone who stutters, the typical reaction is to control the situation, which is the complete opposite of relaxation and softness. The desire for control makes a person who stutters stay physically rigid and mentally alert, constantly preparing for a potential speaking encounter, almost as if bracing for impact. There's also the belief that in order to speak, you have to fight, push and struggle. In this state, even when you're exhausted, you try to stay alert and in control. Ironically, this only leads to more verbal hesitation and blocking.

Aside from the obvious advice of getting more sleep at night, what I suggest is this: do the exact opposite of controlling. Lean into your tiredness – don't fight it. Allow it to guide you and soften you. Focus on your breathing and start going with the flow. It might feel bumpy at first, as you're used to grabbing for control, but as you lean into your tiredness and trust your body to produce speech, you'll begin to see improvement.

> *'Anxiety distorts your personality and makes you unauthentic, forcing you to become someone you aren't. Taking definitive steps to dissolve anxiety awakens your spiritual essence, guiding you back to your true, authentic self. It reconnects you with your deepest inner powers and resources.'*
>
> — Olga Bednarski

Question 51:

Why are we so hard on ourselves for something beyond our control, like a speech impediment? It's not our fault. Despite the challenges, we're unique, smart, talented and kind.

A: Thank you for this thoughtful question. Once again, it highlights the relationship we have with the most important and closest person in our lives – ourselves. No amount of external praise will ever truly suffice or satisfy if a person is experiencing a shortage of love for themselves. Nobody else can do the work of loving us for us – it must come from within us. Each and every one of us.

You're hard on yourself because you don't fully accept yourself, and without acceptance, self-love can't flourish. Self-love isn't about vanity or selfishness; it's about nurturing a supportive and understanding relationship with yourself. It's the foundation upon which everything else in life is built. From this foundation, a new, more peaceful life begins – a life where you're grounded and at ease with yourself, making everything else feel lighter and more manageable. This is where unnecessary suffering ceases.

So often we mistakenly look for love externally, hoping it will fill the void within us. But it doesn't work that way. True self-love isn't something we find outside – it's something we cultivate inside. And as it grows, so does our strength, because the most vital relationship in our lives – the one we have with ourselves – comes into harmony.

Many people in the world struggle with self-love, often because they didn't receive enough of it from their caregivers or parents. But here's the good news: self-love is a skill, and like any skill it can be learned and developed. You can learn to love and appreciate yourself instead of demanding perfection or trying to fit into some predetermined mould to be liked, loved, appreciated or respected. Once you understand that your worth isn't tied to whether someone likes you or how many likes you get on social media, you'll see that external validation offers only fleeting satisfaction. It evaporates quickly, leaving you chasing more.

In contrast, the inner peace that comes from genuine self-acceptance and love is enduring. It's a deeply healing sensation that nourishes and sustains you regardless of what's happening around you. External events – whether successes or setbacks, people coming or going – are transient. But the stillness and strength you find through self-love are lasting. They bring a sense of aliveness and put an end to the exhausting marathon of seeking validation from others.

When you truly love yourself, you begin to see yourself for who you are – your strengths, uniqueness, talents, intelligence and kindness. Without self-love, it's nearly impossible to fully recognize or appreciate these qualities. Self-love is not a luxury; it's the way forward – not just for PWS but for everyone in this world.

Question 52:

How do I deal with the embarrassment and social (un)acceptance of stuttering?

A: The way to deal with this is by changing the way you relate to yourself. Most PWS often have a very limited (narrow) view of themselves, typically seeing themselves only through the lens of their speech. Stop seeing yourself solely through the lens of stuttering and letting it occupy your entire existence. You need to learn to see yourself as more than just someone who stutters. Expand your self-concept, your working theory of yourself, and allow it to reach far beyond stuttering.

There's a lot of debate around the topic of accepting stuttering, with some groups turning into tight-knit sanctuaries where they try to encourage other PWS to accept stuttering as an inherent part of who they are, as just another way of speaking. Some even go so far as to say 'stuttering is beautiful', which, while well-intentioned, is often disconnected from the reality many face. The truth is, speech anxiety causes more than just discomfort; it leads to real suffering for many, interwoven with shame and guilt about having it – feelings that indicate people are far from accepting it. If there were an easy way to simply accept it, we wouldn't still be asking these questions.

As for societal acceptance, we must be realistic. PWS make up less than 2 per cent of the global population. It's unrealistic to expect society to educate every individual on every possible condition, including stuttering. Trying to change the world for you is a losing battle from the start, and our lifetimes are too short to wait for society to evolve.

It's wiser, more practical and far quicker to understand the mechanics of your stuttering, shift your mindset, and learn how to alter your inner speech dynamics at will – much like shifting gears in a car – rather than hoping society will change for you. What's most important in your journey to reclaim your speech and manage embarrassment is self-acceptance. I believe that society will start to accept you – or more accurately, you'll begin to feel more accepted – once you reconcile with and accept yourself. It all starts within you. Don't expect society to accept you if you struggle to accept yourself.

Self-acceptance (reconciliation) is a powerful healing tool. It's an attitude, not a feeling, and can be nurtured in any emotional state or 'speaking experience'. It brings comfort, relieves unnecessary expectations from yourself and others, and can significantly reduce speech anxiety. In fact, with this sense of self-acceptance, you'll find that societal acceptance matters less and less. You'll feel at ease in your own skin, in your own company, and that, in itself, is incredibly freeing. Those who seek societal acceptance often do so because they lack self-acceptance and look to others to fill that void.

True self-acceptance comes from self-discovery – the realization that there is so much more to you than just your stutter. You're multidimensional. Stuttering is just a learned behaviour, a coping strategy that you haven't yet let go of because, subconsciously, it feels safe and familiar.

As you learn more about yourself, you'll become more compassionate and loving towards yourself. Acceptance stems from love. You don't accept people you don't love – you only accept those who matter to you, those you love. So, if you truly intend to accept yourself – whether you stutter or speak fluently – start with love. You might find that, over time, it no longer matters to you as much. As a result of this deeper self-understanding, shifting attitudes and changes in your state of being, your speech anxiety will likely reduce in intensity and may gradually dissipate. This is because your inner states (anxious, calm, kind, etc.) all have physical manifestations.

Do you still feel the need for social acceptance? Keep in mind that no amount of external acceptance will heal the fact that you don't love, or even might hate yourself. That's just another myth. Everything you need is already inside of you.

Question 53:

I believe many people who stutter might avoid group meetings and conversations, not just out of fear of embarrassment, but to avoid making a poor first impression. What are your thoughts on this?

A: Let me start with a few questions: What opinion do you hold of yourself that makes you feel embarrassed or afraid of making a bad first impression? Is it fear of being yourself, a sense of inadequacy or feelings of inferiority? These all point to years of self-criticism and a lack of self-love – patterns of self-abuse that no one deserves to endure.

As I've said before, everything begins with the quality of the relationship you have with yourself. This relationship determines how you feel before entering a situation, how you respond during it and what you anticipate before social encounters even happen.

For PWS, who are often notorious perfectionists (sometimes acutely so), the concern isn't as much about what others say – it's about what *you* say to yourself. What follows is often a cascade of self-critical and undermining thoughts. Sadly, harsh and destructive inner dialogue is not only common among PWS but is also normalised in broader society. For the most severe perfectionists, this inner critic can feel relentless, eating away at their confidence and causing profound inner turmoil. The most painful aspect is that this accusing, critical voice can persist for prolonged periods, creating real suffering and sometimes leading to avoidance of speaking altogether. But avoiding interaction is hardly an effective solution.

The real solution is to silence your inner critic – or, better yet, to change the tone and content of its voice. This transformation begins with fostering a loving, compassionate and healthier relationship with yourself. If you're wondering where to start, take a look at my other responses to similar questions. The key lies in cultivating self-love, something many of us didn't receive enough of during childhood and, as a result, lack in adulthood.

Ask yourself this: Why would you even entertain thoughts of embarrassment or worry about making a negative impression if you were content and accepting of yourself? Why would such concerns even arise? When you anticipate these outcomes, you visualize negative mental images, unconsciously creating the very experiences you fear and making them feel inevitable.

Everything begins and ends with you. You're the centre of your world, and your world – and the experiences within it – exist because of you. You're the source. As unusual as it may sound, there's nothing truly 'outside' of you.

Consider this: every night, as you lie in bed, you're faced with yourself – your thoughts, your narratives and your ideas, ruminating over the past or projecting into the future. No one else can step into this inner world to alter it, to make you feel better, to force you, to criticise or to praise you. This world is entirely yours. You're its sole dweller and its master.

And here's the most profound truth: You have the power to create either hell or paradise within your inner world. The choice lies in the relationship you cultivate with yourself. It can either nourish or deplete you, depending on your ability to step back from the hypnotizing projections of the mind and its often-harsh narratives.

The quality of your social relationships is deeply connected to the quality of the relationship you have with yourself. Everything stems from that foundation.

Question 54:

Why do people often respond with laughter or irritation to stuttering, even though everyone makes speech mistakes, and no one is perfect? Shouldn't empathy, rather than ridicule, be the response, as we all face judgment or hurtful comments in our own lives?

A: Empathy from others becomes possible when you first extend empathy, support and understanding to yourself. Wouldn't you agree that no one would dare ridicule someone who radiates calmness, confidence and unconditional self-acceptance? Ridicule, even when unintentional, often targets those who see themselves as victims and struggle with self-rejection – whether it's because of stuttering or any other perceived flaw.

People subconsciously sense and mirror back what we project. When we carry self-loathing or a lack of self-acceptance, it can feel unattractive, even inviting latent aggression or discomfort from others. If you want empathy from others, it begins with learning to give it to yourself first. Start by noticing how you speak to yourself (your inner dialogue) – what you say and how you react when things don't go as planned or when you make mistakes.

Learning the art of self-love is a journey, but one worth taking. When you embrace and accept yourself fully, you stop being at odds with yourself and become your own ally. This shift within transforms your inner state, leaving you feeling empowered and nourished. People will sense this transformation, too.

When you start liking yourself, you naturally become more open, genuine and uninhibited. You stop editing yourself and simply show up as the real you. This inner change sparks a noticeable shift in how others respond to you. At first, it might surprise you – or even feel unfamiliar – but soon it will become your new normal.

Do yourself a favour: learn to love yourself and always stand by your side. Expecting others to change their attitudes or behaviour before you can feel satisfied is a futile and frustrating path. True growth begins with you because you're the only person within your control, and you're the closest one to yourself.

Self-love and compassion aren't just abstract concepts from a book – they are attitudes you can cultivate and live every day. With intention and practice, they can become your constant companions, transforming your experience of life.

Question 55:

I've stuttered since I was a kid and still do at 41. I hate it and feel embarrassed by others who stutter too. My communication skills are poor; I confuse words and struggle to explain myself, leading me to want to hide. I've missed job and relationship opportunities because I avoid talking and explaining things. How can I accept my disability?

A: It pains me to hear about your suffering and how it's causing you to miss out on so much of what life has to offer. I sense that you're hoping that 'accepting your disability' might ease your struggles and bring you peace. But that belief, too, is an illusion. If living a reclusive, restricted life isn't your ideal vision, adopting this label might only deepen your sense of limitation and despair.

The term 'disability' is rarely applicable to most cases of stuttering – except in instances tied to physical causes like cranial damage, blood clots or strokes. For most, it risks becoming a self-imposed restriction, a mental straitjacket. And as we know, straitjackets are suffocating.

If you truly want to move beyond this, the way forward lies in becoming aware of how you unconsciously create the experience of anxiety and stuttering. Awareness is key to loosening the grip these patterns have on your life. From there, you can begin to disidentify from them – gradually but decisively taking daily steps towards a life where these struggles no longer control you.

One cannot live by avoiding life.

Question 56:

How do you, as a stutterer, handle dating?

A: Dating can be a challenging journey for many PWS, and I've often heard it's especially so for men, who are traditionally expected to be more assertive in initiating contact and showing interest.

The key lies in how you approach dating. Many PWS focus heavily on their stuttering, often trying to hide it at all costs. But this strategy can backfire, increasing stress and tension, making it nearly impossible to relax and exude natural confidence. On top of that, you may find yourself overly focused on achieving a specific outcome – whether that's landing a date or a more intimate goal. No judgment here; we all have different intentions.

However, when you become tense and nervous, your natural response is often to close off emotionally. You may unconsciously adopt a protective or defensive posture, which reflects in your body language. This can send signals that conflict with your desire to connect. Remember, dating is ultimately about creating an intimate connection with another person. To do that, you need to take certain emotional risks, be a little vulnerable and allow your heart to open.

That can feel scary, right? The risk of emotional exposure might seem overwhelming. To reduce that sense of risk, I suggest letting go of rigid expectations before any dating experience. Don't approach it with the mindset of 'I must meet someone tonight'. Instead, have an open-ended scenario for your evening and shift your focus to enjoying the moment and the interactions themselves.

Consider turning these occasions into opportunities to build and refine your social skills – your personal 'training ground' where you can experiment, make mistakes, show your quirks, play and learn. When you treat these situations as playful rather than pressured, the stakes immediately feel lower, and you become freer to explore. Leave space for the universe (God, fate or whatever resonates with you) to guide you to the right person. Do not force anything. Trust in the process while embracing playfulness. It's a skill that takes time to develop, but it's worth the effort. After all, we've all spent years learning unhelpful habits; now is the time to learn effective and empowering ones.

Finally, here's something I want to leave you with: whether you're a man or a woman, if you feel and act as though you're already loved, you'll never truly be alone. Don't just take my word for it – test it out for yourself. If it doesn't work, your shell will still be there waiting for you. But what if it does work? Imagine the possibilities: a different life, one that's easier, lighter and filled with connection.

Question 57:

I've noticed that my stuttering often stems from the fear of speaking and overthinking others' opinions. When I'm alone or with close friends and family, like my siblings, I stutter much less or not at all. However, speaking to strangers or in front of a camera, especially in public speaking, overwhelms me with thoughts about others' reactions rather than focusing on what I'm saying.

You might suggest calming down and accepting it, but it's not that simple. How did you manage the mental aspects of stuttering?

A: The core reason for your struggle ultimately lies in how you relate to and react to yourself when your speaking performance falls below your expectations. Even before entering a social situation, you've already set certain standards for how you *must* speak to feel acceptable or 'good enough' in your own eyes. Your greatest fear isn't necessarily how others will react, but rather how *you* will react to yourself. Deep down, you carry the belief that you're somehow 'flawed' or 'not good enough', which turns social experiences into struggles – where you constantly strive to conceal your perceived imperfections and seek validation.

When you speak to family members or when you're alone, your grip on yourself naturally loosens. There are no rigid standards to comply with, no pressure to meet expectations – allowing your speech to flow effortlessly. In these moments, the tension (i.e. both mental and physical resistance) eases, and you experience the fluency that has always been within you.

People come and go; they don't dwell on your speech. But when they leave, what remains is you – your thoughts, your inner dialogue and that critical, even bullying, voice inside your head. And so, once again, we return to the core issue – your relationship with yourself. Take a closer look. Listen to the way you habitually speak to yourself. What messages are you repeating? Consider writing them down and replacing them with words that uplift and support you, rather than drown you in self-doubt and insecurities.

Criticism and self-judgment never lead to growth or improvement in any area of life. Harshness only causes you to close off from yourself and the world, creating feelings of isolation and disconnection that lead to suffering. Let go of the need for self-criticism and rigid expectations – this too is a choice you can make. Next time you stumble or even block, choose to refrain from your habitual inner castigations and say something kindly compassionate and show to yourself that you are indeed on your side. You'll see a tremendous change in your state of being, almost like a gratitude filling you up from inside.

I can almost hear you thinking, *'But my negativity is based on real past experiences… this always happens to me.'*

Here's what I want you to remember – your past is just a story you keep telling yourself. It defines you only to the extent that you allow it to. You have the power to create a new relationship with yourself – one that's not dictated by the past but inspired by the future you desire. Don't let yesterday's experiences limit who you can become today. It's a conscious choice, and you have the ability to make it, starting right now. When you do, your social experiences – and your life – will begin to transform in ways you never imagined.

True acceptance is the key to finding inner peace. But what does real acceptance mean? It's not about giving up or resigning yourself to stuttering; rather, it's about releasing the fight and embracing a neutral stance. Acceptance means acknowledging where you are right now while knowing that you have the intention to change. It feels liberating and nourishing – not passive or resigned.

With the right mindset and a step-by-step approach, you can gently peel away the layers of self-doubt and replace them with fresh, life-affirming beliefs and ideas. Over the coming months of regular application, you'll find yourself stepping into greater confidence, fluency and ease – one step at a time.

Question 58:

I'm having a really bad day. I just started a great new job, but my stutter is making things hard. I feel defeated, and I'm afraid if I tell my boss, they'll think I'm not fit for the job. My frustration is making my stutter even worse, and I've developed a tick where I bite myself when I stutter. Everything hurts, and I feel so useless. How did you handle it?

A: You're struggling with intense self-hatred, even punishing yourself through self-harm, like biting. I too once suffered, from compulsive skin-picking, which was my way of torturing myself. The key to healing is reconciliation with yourself through self-love. I know this advice may sound repetitive, but I've never been more certain of anything in my life than the transformative power of self-love. It's a nurturing force that brings incredible benefits to all areas of your life – mind, body and spirit. But remember, its true power comes from practice, not just reading about it. I encourage you to try it without delay and experience the profound changes for yourself.

Practical techniques and strategies for fluency

Question 59:

I had a rough day with my speech, struggled to speak and felt frustrated and quiet afterward. What strategies help you cope with bad speech days?

A: When you started experiencing turbulence, what thoughts came to mind? What did you say to yourself? Typically, PWS tend to catastrophize and be quite unforgiving towards themselves, making the situation even harder. The more you emotionally invest in negativity (e.g. a speech block), the more turbulence you'll experience.

The Gentle Strategy: What I recommend is that, before starting each day, you forgive yourself sincerely and from the heart. Give yourself permission to make mistakes and be imperfect. Sit with your self-acceptance and notice what feelings arise. If you approach this with sincerity, you may experience a sense of expansion in your chest (your heart area) and a general lightness throughout your body, as though a weight has fallen from your shoulders.

The compulsion to be perfect and the constant effort to maintain control can feel incredibly heavy. With self-forgiveness, you'll approach situations with fewer expectations and less pressure, and your speech might even improve from the very first attempt. On turbulent days, sincere self-forgiveness helps you let go of 'bad days' more easily – without agonizing over them – so you can move forward. If you dwell on your 'bad speaking performance', you reinforce and intensify the problem. I explore 'the aftermath' in more detail in my book *The Anatomy of Stuttering* (Bednarski, 2022).

If we look deeper at this situation – taking a broader view – we see this once again leads back to self-love and your relationship with yourself.

Here's another strategy: imagine for a moment that it was your child having a difficult speaking day, or perhaps someone you deeply admire sharing how challenging their day had been. What would you say to them? I'm sure you would find kind and supportive words to reassure them, encourage them and lift their spirits. You would remind them that it's not the end of the world, right?

So why not offer that same kindness to yourself? Why not become a compassionate and supportive friend to yourself?

I know self-support isn't something most of us have been conditioned to practise, but perhaps it's time to learn. Become that best friend to yourself – the one who is always on your side.

Question 60:

Have you tried SpeechEasy (assistive technology)? If so, would you recommend it?

A: I don't have personal experience of using such devices, but I believe they could be helpful for short-term use. However, relying on technology for constant and prolonged use may not be the best approach. From what I've observed, people who purchase these devices often fall into the trap of hoping the technology will cure their stuttering, or they begin to rely on it as a constant companion in their interactions. This is where the issue arises – it can lead to disappointment and frustration because, while the tech can assist, it cannot cure.

What I've also noticed is that once someone buys one device, they don't usually stop there. They often continue trying different ones, hoping to find the one that will 'cure' their stutter, but without success.

In my view, it's easier and more empowering to shift your mindset and learn to regulate the inner dynamics of your speech to restore fluency. Instead of trying every device available, you can work on expressing yourself naturally, even if that means occasional stumbles and embracing being 'perfectly imperfect'. What most PWS truly desire is the ability to communicate fully and freely, without becoming dependent on assistive technology.

Devices focus only on the superficial manifestation of stuttering, and while they may seem like an easy fix for some, they can mask who you really are. I believe they take away the opportunity to discover your true voice, to unlock it and to fall in love with it.

At the end of the day, when you want to tell someone you love them, you wouldn't want a robotic voice to say those words for you, would you? You would want to say them yourself.

Remember, all the answers are already within you.

'There is no way to separate speech from personality and study it in isolation. How well we speak is always context-dependent – shaped by the situations we find ourselves in, the people we interact with, and how we think, perceive and feel in those moments. To truly understand stuttering and its inner workings, we must look beyond speech alone. We need to explore the broader factors within our worldview that shape our experiences and contribute to the problem.'

— Olga Bednarski

Question 61:

Do you think practising the letters you stammer on can help reduce or smooth out the stutter?

A: I don't believe this approach helps, at least not in the long term. When you focus solely on practising letters, you're addressing only the speech-related aspects of the challenge while completely overlooking the psychological side. Practising letters often comes with the hope that you won't stutter, but ironically, the harder you practise, the more effortful and challenging speaking can become – leading to frustration and all the familiar feelings that come with it.

Instead, try to look beyond the stuttering. Don't make a big deal out of the letters or give any particular letter a 'VIP' status. Shift your focus to the person behind the speech – yourself.

Question 62:

Are there any vocal exercises to help with stuttering?

A: Yes, there are many techniques to try, but one of my all-time favourites is called 'The Cork'. For this exercise, you place a cork from a wine bottle gently between your front teeth and begin reading aloud. Just a couple of minutes of fully engaged reading can work wonders – it helps open up your throat, loosen your glottal and vocal cords, and improve both your vocal pitch and pronunciation, leaving your speech clearer and more resonant than before.

A little tip: keep a napkin handy – you might need it to catch a bit of saliva while you practise!

Question 63:

I've noticed that I stutter less if I clench my teeth while speaking. It also makes my throat feel more relaxed, whereas I usually get sore pain in my lower tongue or upper throat. Speaking with my teeth clenched seems easier. Can you explain why this might be?

A: Here's a gentle way to reframe your understanding: it's essentially a trick to shift your mind's focus. For instance, clenching your teeth redirects your attention, much like intentionally pulling your ear might do. By focusing on the discomfort caused by such an action, you may notice an improvement in fluency.

Many PWS go to great lengths to avoid or control their stutter. However, I suggest a kinder, more effective approach: instead of fighting against it, cultivate awareness of how you may unintentionally contribute to the issue. Gradually, replace unhelpful habits with behaviours that foster ease and flow in your speech.

One day, you'll wake up and find yourself wondering what all the fuss was about. You'll look back and realize how much energy was spent dwelling on stuttering when your journey could have been one of learning, self-compassion and growth instead.

Question 64:

How do you break out of the cycle of overthinking and negative self-talk?

A: Here's how:

- Find a quiet place where you can be with yourself. If you're in a busy workplace, even a public toilet cubicle will work – any place where you can have a moment of peace.
- Clearly identify the thoughts that are troubling you. Take a sheet of paper and a pen and write them down. This will help you see the internal dialogue you're having. Look at it, really see it.
- Ask yourself, 'Is this the kind of dialogue I want to continue in my mind? Does it support me, or does it undermine me?'
- Choose new thoughts that you want to think and start thinking them on purpose. Say them to yourself on purpose. For example, to calm yourself and uplift your spirits, you might say things like, 'I'm safe, I'm supported, I'm protected, my opinion matters, I'm loved, I love myself, life is guiding me towards the best resolution for my problems,' and so on.
- Write your chosen new thoughts (ideas) down. Read them and repeat them in your mind until the negative talk stops and you feel better and more positive. You can write down as many new thoughts as you need. Consider carrying a small notebook with you so you can remind yourself before important events, like job interviews, dates or any social interactions.

Most importantly: do it! Reading about it alone won't help. Apply this technique and watch the results unfold. Practise regularly (at least three months) and you'll gradually banish negative, toxic and undermining thought patterns.

In their place, you'll cultivate kind, peaceful and supportive inner conversations. This transformation will lead to amazing results in all areas of your life – speech, social life, career, love life and beyond.

Question 65:

Will consistent practising of speech techniques bring me closer to achieving fluency?

A: It's unlikely that speech techniques alone will lead to lasting change. These techniques often focus on the speech itself and its perceived deficiencies. Many PWS who rely on these methods fall into the trap of striving for speech perfection, constantly monitoring their performance and anxiously waiting for results. This mindset can be counterproductive and actually takes you further from achieving fluency. It's like trying to chase a horizontal line that seems to move further away the closer you get.

Instead, look beyond speech, beyond the surface symptoms and focus on the root of the issue. The guidance you need on how to do this is found within the pages of this guidebook.

Alternatively, consider combining speech techniques with inner work. Make that inner work a priority – it's just as essential in your journey to healing.

Question 66:

What are your thoughts about using a text-to-speech phone app in daily life? I've been going through a tough period where my stuttering has been worse than it's been in years. Stuttering constantly is physically and mentally exhausting, and dealing with people's reactions – like that instinctive, involuntary laughter – can be emotionally draining.

This got me thinking about using a phone app for communication. Since most people have their phones with them, why not use an app when needed? I'm curious if the tech is already out there and functional, and how well it works in real-life situations, like ordering a coffee at Starbucks. How do people react, and can these apps keep up with the pace of normal conversation?

A: My first thought is that using this app could become an obstacle in itself, as it may feel unnatural and awkward. This is especially true since you're already concerned about how others might perceive you using it. Additionally, you know that you can speak well in certain non-pressured situations, and this only makes it more uncomfortable to suddenly pull out your phone and let an app speak for you.

There are many apps available now, and some might be helpful to a certain extent, especially for online interactions. However, for face-to-face conversations, I believe they can create an even greater sense of discomfort and awkwardness. After all, people want to talk to you – the unique individual – not a soulless robotic app. Wouldn't you agree?

All these external solutions, like magic tricks, may act like anaesthetics – temporarily numbing the pain but not truly removing it.

Once again, I want to emphasize that it's easier to understand speech anxiety, get to know yourself on a deeper level and gradually dissolve it. In doing so, you can free yourself from daily fear, anxiety and exhaustion. The solution is much closer than you might think – it's already within you right now. It's faster and more effective than enduring all the discomfort and awkwardness of using various apps for something so natural that you can do yourself.

Don't run away from yourself. Start running towards yourself. The results will surpass your expectations.

Question 67:

Has anyone else found that juggling objects while speaking helps to eliminate their stutter?

A: Juggling serves as a powerful attention distractor, much like how pulling your ears while speaking – say, during a phone call – can temporarily reduce or even eliminate stuttering. If you're sceptical, I encourage you to test this for yourself. Don't just take my word for it – explore, experiment and discover what works for you.

Support systems and external influences

Question 68:

My old friend at work noticed that my stammer has improved significantly. He asked if I was attending speech classes, and I said no. Even with him accompanied by two people I didn't know, I spoke freely and even shared a joke. I'm happy with this change and no longer try to hide my stammer. What might be causing this improvement?

A: You feel good, you speak well.

Speech anxiety is influenced by the level of emotional and psychological comfort you experience in each situation, often even before you begin speaking. Your emotional comfort sets the tone for your state of being (or state of mind). Typically, when you're in a flow, there's a sense of inner comfort and, as a result, there's no resistance, no mental rehearsals and no attempts to control your self-expression – your speech. With your inner dynamics in harmony, you flow effortlessly and easily. When you stop controlling, when you let go, as John Harrison puts it, you stop interfering with the intricate process that's meant to be automatic and effortless. And as a result, you flow.

However, when emotional discomfort and physical tension enter the equation, the situation becomes more challenging – even if the circumstances are the same or similar.

So, what causes this fluctuation in fluency, and why does it come in waves? It all comes down to your inner dynamics and how they function in different situations, life stages and moments. When these dynamics are in harmony, your speech flows effortlessly. But when they're out of sync, you may struggle and block – even without emotional anxiety.

Speech is a dynamic process. Think of it like building with Lego blocks – there are different parts, but what you get depends on how you arrange them. You have all the individual components, but how they work together in your brain depends on factors such as attention, breathing patterns, muscle tension, intention, attitude, habits, beliefs and many others.

The good news is that all of these elements are changeable, just like Lego blocks – once you become aware of how they work. For you, these changes may occur from one situation to another and at different times in your life, especially during certain experiences or shifts in belief. You can consciously redesign and adjust your speech dynamics once you understand how all the individual blocks involved in the speaking process operate.

My advice is this: when you notice an improvement in your fluency, acknowledge your ability to stay fluid. At the same time, treat it as the norm – don't get overly excited about it. You may wonder why. Overexcitement often indicates underlying psychological discomfort, which stems from the novelty of the fluency experience. Whenever something makes us uncomfortable, we tend to shy away from it and return to the familiarity of our previous state – even if that state is uncomfortable. Familiarity feels safer, even if it's not ideal, because it's predictable. This all happens unconsciously, so you might not even be aware of it.

Relate to your improvement as just part of the norm. Breathe out, enjoy it and know that as your mind is in a state of flow, you can broaden your perspective about yourself. Recognize how multidimensional you are and how much life has to offer once you free yourself from focusing solely on stuttering and speech-related concerns. You can look beyond stuttering.

Question 69:

I've tried various courses for people who stutter, but none seem to work. Why don't these courses work, and how can I avoid feeling like a failure or irresponsible?

A: Do not blame yourself – this is not your fault. You're doing your best to help yourself, and that's truly commendable. I suspect that the courses you've tried so far have focused mainly on one aspect of stuttering: the speech itself. Most programmes out there tend to overlook the psychological aspect because they either don't see the connection or aren't sure how to address it.

I encourage you to explore alternative approaches, like the one discussed in this book. With the abundance of advice I've already shared, you can even begin this journey on your own. However, if you feel you need guidance, don't hesitate to reach out and ask for help. Also, be sure to check out my explanatory videos on my YouTube channel, 'Stop Stuttering with Olga'.

Question 70:

I feel that nothing can help me overcome stuttering and often question new methodologies and sceptical towards ex-stutterers who offer help. I worry that they haven't truly experienced stuttering and are just seeking to profit. Why is this the case?

A: Whenever I hear someone say that nothing and no one can help them, I sense a strong sense of ego or pride holding them back. It tries to convince them that they and their impediment are so uniquely special that they might as well keep it. This mindset prevents people from opening their hearts to the help and support that's available, and from exploring other options. There may also be some resentment from past experiences where you reached out for help, only to be turned away, often by those closest to us.

I encourage you to take the emotional risk of opening your heart. Let go of the rationalizations and reach out for support. Ask, and you shall receive. It may feel uncomfortable at first, and that's completely normal – it's part of learning something new. Don't be discouraged by the initial discomfort, because it won't last long.

Something tells me that most former stutterers are more than willing to help, as this was once our source of suffering too. I remember when I first started, I provided guidance for free. My channel is always here for you, whenever you need it.

Career and public speaking challenges

Question 71:

Should I discuss my stuttering in my personal statement when applying for a highly competitive study programme? I've heard conflicting advice: some say disclosing a disability can led to negative judgments or misunderstandings, while others suggest it can highlight resilience.

A: My perspective on this is that you should begin by asking yourself two important questions: How would I feel if I included this in my personal statement? And how would I feel if I didn't disclose it but briefly mentioned it just before the interview? Whatever choice you make, ensure it comes from a place of positive intention and certainty – free from second-guessing or regrets later on. Be confident in your decision and, once you've made it, follow through without looking back.

When discussing it, I believe negative judgments or misunderstandings are more likely if it's shared with an apologetic tone, as though you're inconveniencing others by having this aspect of your life. On the other hand, if you approach it with a neutral yet confident tone, framing it as a unique trait that contributes to who you are, the response is likely to be neutral or even positive. In fact, as you mentioned, it can highlight your resilience and inner strength of character.

People often pick up on the feelings and attitudes with which we communicate, even when it's through writing. That's why it's important to package your message with positive, or at least neutral, energy. Avoid writing about yourself in an apologetic tone or while feeling angry or resentful. Additionally, as a former HR graduate, I would advise against going into too much detail – especially since some readers may not have the expertise to fully understand it. A brief mention will suffice.

In summary, this is a deeply personal decision, and there isn't a definitive right or wrong answer. Trust your own judgment. If including it feels right and won't lead to overthinking or regrets later, then go ahead and include it. If it feels uncomfortable, or you think you might agonize over it afterwards, it's perfectly okay to leave it out. Ultimately, it's about what feels best for you and aligns with your peace of mind.

Question 72:

How do you handle someone who constantly finishes your sentences? I politely asked them to stop, but now I feel guilty for setting that boundary. Any advice on addressing this and starting a constructive conversation?

A: The only way to handle situations like this is to express yourself openly – people can't read your mind. And that's exactly what you've done. Be fully on your own side in such moments; this will help dissolve feelings of guilt, inadequacy and shame. If you're not on your side, you're likely to feel wrong for standing up for yourself, as if you've committed some kind of offence.

But here's the truth: you have nothing to feel guilty about. You stood up for yourself, set clear boundaries and should be proud of that. Imagine if a stranger walked into your home and started taking your belongings. If you stood up to them and protected what was yours, would you feel guilty? Of course not! You have every right to protect what's important to you and ask them to leave.

The same principle applies to speaking situations. If someone crosses your boundaries or behaves in a way that upsets you, the appropriate response is to address it. Let them know what's unacceptable and what you need from them. That's how you assert yourself and protect your emotional space.

If you want the conversation to flow more constructively, you could pre-emptively let the other person know what you need. For instance, if you're naturally a slower speaker or anticipate challenges, you might kindly say something like, 'I'd really appreciate it if you could be patient, let me finish my sentences and avoid interrupting.' This is a polite and constructive way to set expectations, but make sure to say it firmly and with confidence so they know you mean it.

Most importantly, don't expect people to guess what you're thinking – let them know clearly. And remember, don't second-guess your actions. You've done an excellent job setting boundaries and standing up for yourself. That's something to celebrate! Give yourself a big hug – you deserve it.

Question 73:

Although my stuttering has improved, I still get nervous about saying names. I avoid introducing people for fear of messing up their names. Tonight, I introduced one friend but froze on the second friend's name, and she had to say it herself. I felt foolish. Why do I get nervous about names, and how can I break this cycle?

A: This happens because *you're performing* – viewing the situation through a negative lens (anticipating failure) and visualizing yourself struggling even before the event arises. As a result, you avoid and fear these situations, literally setting yourself up for failure before they even occur. You don't realize you're doing this; it's unconscious. But now that you're aware, you have the power to change your reactions and intentions. You can intentionally shift your mindset and approach these situations like a star at a social gathering.

Instead of performing, which creates stress, increases tension and triggers the fear of social failure (even to the point of imagining it's a life-or-death scenario), try seeing the situation for what it truly is: a fun social event with friends. The only person demanding perfection and terrorizing themselves with fear is you. Let go of the performance mindset, stop attaching an exaggerated significance to the situation and start having fun. When you switch to having fun and see the event for what it is, you'll become more relatable, natural and spontaneous. Fun and humour will dissolve the unnecessary seriousness your mind attaches to the situation.

Since you see these events as a performance where you expect to be judged negatively, you're looking at them through a negative lens. What you focus on expands, making the situation seem harder, with higher stakes and riskier. The antidote to this distorted perception is to intentionally view the event as a fun social gathering, nothing more. Also, check in with yourself: do you tend to look for the bad, or do you look for the good in situations? Choose to focus on the good. Remind yourself that this is your opportunity to socialize, enjoy and have fun. Make this your central focus. Right now, it seems like the only thing on your mind when introducing your friends is the pressure of the moment, blocking out the fact that you're meeting friends to have fun. Shift your focus back to the joy of connection and friendship. That should become your priority.

The third practical tip: start intentionally imagining (visualizing) yourself making social introductions with ease, without hesitation. As long as you hold on to the image of yourself blocking, fearing and avoiding these situations, you'll continue to experience anxiety, fearful anticipation and avoidance, followed by feelings of shame or foolishness afterwards. Your invisible behaviour – your thoughts and visualizations of social failure – becomes your visible experience of blocking.

If you want to reduce, or even eliminate, these situations, choose an alternative scenario. Begin visualizing yourself in these situations, remaining fluid, open, confident and unapologetic – having fun introducing others rather than avoiding these moments.

Question 74:

I'm nervous I might stutter during the interview. How can I manage my nerves?

A: Before entering any situation, it's important to honestly and sincerely forgive yourself for any potential blunders, stumbles or imperfections. This might sound like an odd practice to some, but I don't mind how it sounds. If you do it with intention, it brings a sense of liberation and significantly eases anxiety and perfectionism.

Visualize yourself speaking confidently and fluently during the interview. To make sure this isn't just wishful thinking, you must tap into the feelings of what it would truly be like to speak without stuttering. Feelings make your visualization real, and as you feel it in your body, you begin to rehearse for success. Often, PWS unknowingly rehearse for failure, becoming masters of terrorizing themselves. Instead, consciously rehearse success, training your mind and body to flow more naturally and comfortably. Remember, control doesn't come from force; it comes from ease and flow. Use the power of your imagination the same way you might use it to evoke nervousness or anxiety – only this time, flip it to invite calm and confidence.

Don't cling to this job opportunity as if it's the last one in the world. The more you desire it too desperately, the more tension and fear you create around losing it. And you probably already know what tends to happen when we desperately cling to something or fear losing it. According to the law of attraction, by constantly thinking and worrying about what you don't want to happen (like losing a job), you're actually inviting that very scenario into your life. It's the law of resonance in action.

Instead, practise detachment from the outcome. Let go of expectations or fantasies about how things might unfold. Ideally, it would help if you could reconcile with the possibility that you might not get the job – confronting that fear before it even arises. This will help reduce the excitement and anxiety associated with big hopes, creating inner steadiness and balance. As a result, you'll appear more natural and competent because you're not attached to the outcome, nor trying to control the situation. When we expect something, we become rigid and attempt to control external events or people, which only leads to disappointment, frustration and suffering.

One of my 'secret' tricks is what I call modelling the situation in advance. Write down, on paper (yes, by hand), how you would like the situation to unfold. Be specific about how you want to feel emotionally and physically – your state of being. Writing by hand helps you connect with yourself more deeply, free from digital distractions. The more details you include, the more real it becomes. Once you've described your own experience of the situation, imagine the experience of the person (or people) you're meeting. How do they feel while interacting with you? Approach this exercise with gratitude and positivity. One key thing: don't focus on the final outcome. Let it unfold naturally.

Most importantly, reflect on and apply everything above. Just reading about it won't magically change your situation. The real change comes from taking action.

Question 75:

Two months ago, an interviewer laughed at my stutter, and I didn't get the job. This, along with other hurtful comments, has left me feeling depressed and scared. I have another interview coming up and want to feel confident. How can I overcome these past experiences and not let them affect me? Please advise.

A: Your feelings are completely valid, and I'm deeply saddened by the fact that you were laughed at. I truly feel for you. However, don't let these past negative experiences define your future or rob you of your chances for success. I believe this goal can be achieved through a therapeutic approach that offers a fresh perspective on situations, helping you to no longer invest emotionally in such moments.

Here's my practical therapeutic advice. First, realize and accept that the majority of fluent speakers have never encountered stuttering in their lives. They might have only a vague understanding of what it is, and therefore their reactions are often born from ignorance. Impulsive laughter is typically a sign of their own discomfort or embarrassment, not a reflection of you. It's important to recognize that they simply don't know how to respond appropriately.

With this understanding, choose not to take their behaviour personally (unless, of course, you're subjected to abuse or name-calling). Instead, consciously cultivate feelings of compassion for them, perhaps even pity, recognizing that they are simply unaware, like ill-mannered children. This shift allows you to psychologically step away from the role of a fearful victim, and instead place yourself in a mature, empowered position. You're no longer at the mercy of others' reactions; you're in control. This is a mental exercise of consciously elevating yourself above their ignorance.

This doesn't mean that you should become overbearing or patronizing, as you may fear. Quite the opposite – it positions you as an equal to your listener (for instance, your interviewer), rather than inferior because you stutter.

In fact, you can even choose to make direct, prolonged eye contact, a firm gaze that signals you're a dignified, worthy individual, regardless of who you're speaking to. By doing so, you convey that you mean business, and that you'll stand up for yourself. You're not to be disrespected. Prepare to make them feel uncomfortable for their ignorance – and enjoy doing so.

People will unconsciously sense your inner strength and dignity. When they perceive you as strong and unshaken, it becomes much harder for them to laugh at you or make derogatory remarks. How you emotionally and psychologically position yourself in these situations is key. If you present yourself as an apologetic victim, others will, in all likelihood, treat you as such.

Make this mental exercise part of your preparation before and during these interactions. As you continue to practise this mindset, you'll no longer feel like a victim of passive aggression or external judgment. The reactions of others will no longer affect you and, most likely, they'll stop occurring altogether. You'll feel triumphant.

Remember, don't define yourself solely as someone who stutters. You're so much more than that, and you can reclaim control over your life. Expand your self-concept beyond just being a PWS.

Ultimately, forgive others for their ignorance, and laugh it off. You deserve to be free of this burden.

'If you trust your own opinion, you won't quiver or freeze when expressing it.'

— Olga Bednarski

Question 76:

I'm feeling nervous this morning about my PhD dissertation proposal defence. I need to present on a complex approach, and I pre-recorded the presentation because I struggle with blocking and stammering during live presentations. While some might advise against this, I believe pre-recording helps convey my message clearly. I'll still discuss questions with the committee in the Zoom meeting. What are your thoughts on this approach?

A: I suggest trying an exercise called *modelling* to prepare for your presentation. This simple yet powerful practice allows you to mentally set the tone for how you want a speaking situation to unfold before it happens. To do this exercise, you'll need some paper, a pen and a bit of quiet time.

Start a day or two before your presentation or meeting. Sit down and write, in the past tense, about how you want the interaction to go – whether it's a one-on-one meeting, a group presentation at work, a date or any other context. Imagine that the situation has already taken place, and now you're reflecting on it, describing how you felt psychologically and how you spoke during that moment.

As you write, focus on describing your emotional state in detail. How comfortable did you feel during the situation? Did you deliver your message with ease and confidence? How did you feel physically – was there any tension, compulsion to rush or nervousness like sweaty palms or shaky hands? How was your breathing? Where was your focus during your talk? Did you feel relaxed and present? Be as thorough as you can, and always write as if the event has already happened.

Next, shift your perspective to your listener's point of view. Imagine how they felt during the interaction and write from their perspective. For example: 'I really enjoyed talking to [Your Name]. They seemed so confident and professional. It's clear they are highly knowledgeable in their field, and they made a wonderful impression.'

If you're preparing for a group presentation, describe the audience's reactions in detail. Visualize their facial expressions, their engagement, perhaps even applause or other positive feedback. Imagine the overall impression they had of you and write it down as vividly as possible.

Modelling is most effective when you apply it to any important interaction – job interviews, meetings, presentations or dates. The key is to practise this a day or two before the actual event.

'Overcoming stuttering is about becoming more authentically yourself. It's a journey of gradually shedding outdated ideas and shifting your perceptions – about yourself, others, and life itself.'

— Olga Bednarski

Question 77:

How do you handle the embarrassment of stuttering in public? Recently, while saying grace at a dinner with my church family, I got stuck and stuttered badly. I felt so embarrassed I wanted to leave. How do you manage such situations?

A: With love and self-forgiveness. It's not the event itself, but how you respond to it based on your self-perception and your relationship with yourself. As I mentioned in the previous answer, it's essential to learn to see yourself as greater than your stuttering – to see beyond it – and keep your focus on the entirety of who you are. Getting to know yourself better is the first step towards freedom from anxiety, mastering self-regulation and speaking with ease.

At the moment, you may judge your worth based on how your speech goes. On a bad speech day, you might feel worthless and ashamed, wanting to hide away. On a good speech day, you thrive – but only temporarily – until the next social interaction causes you to fall back into the pit of shame, guilt and self-blame.

The not-so-secret 'secret' to managing these situations in the future is to evolve your relationship with yourself and shift your perception beyond stuttering and speech-related aspects of your identity. As long as your attention remains fixed on speech, you can't see beyond it. Your perspective on the other important parts of your personality remains limited, and you remain stuck in a mind-constructed prison, with stuttering as your only insidious inmate.

Once your relationship with yourself begins to evolve – becoming more supportive, understanding and loving (rather than judgmental, critical and self-punishing) – your inner dialogue will follow suit. Even in the face of challenging situations, your inner voice will be kind and compassionate. Your emotional state will gradually shift to reflect this new way of treating and relating to yourself. You'll notice that you're more willing to come out of your protective shell, becoming more relaxed, natural and spontaneous. You'll feel more comfortable taking emotional risks, presenting your authentic self to others rather than an edited version, knowing that, no matter the outcome or feedback from others, you'll always support yourself.

Your inner dialogue will become benevolent, with a tone that's kind and forgiving. The harshest critic you fear isn't other people – it's what you say to yourself and how you react to yourself in and after these situations. Nobody told you to leave because you stuttered; you told yourself you weren't worthy of being around others. You almost left because you believed you didn't belong. What is this, if not a desire to punish yourself, rooted in a lack of self-love and compassion?

The experience of stuttering begins long before you enter a speaking situation; it's rehearsed in your mind well in advance of any social event. These rehearsals are fuelled by your thoughts, feelings, inner dialogue and the narratives you tell yourself. The blocks that happen in the situation are simply the culmination of all that has been building up prior to the event.

Change the 'how' (how you see and relate to yourself), and you change the 'what' (the situation and its outcome). In other words, by changing how you view and think about yourself, you change what shows up in the world around you.

As Dr Fred Wolf discusses in *The Eagle's Quest*, the observer effect suggests that what you perceive not only affects you but also influences the object of your perception.

At the end of the book, you'll find a practical guide on exactly how to practise self-love – and, importantly, how not to practise it.

***

The greatest challenge for most PWS is that they chronically struggle to see beyond their stuttering – or perhaps they simply refuse to. They focus on one small, acquired aspect of their personality, and become mesmerized by superficial symptoms like blocks, stumbles and hesitations. They fully identify with stuttering and become completely absorbed in these symptoms, obsessively preoccupied with finding ways to 'fix' them, often hoping for a quick and easy solution, like a one-time exercise or practice.

The main objective in overcoming this challenge is to shift your attention away from the mechanics of speech and intentionally look beyond stuttering. This allows you to begin noticing the deeper dynamics of your personality and behaviours that are keeping you stuck in the cycle of stuttering. The goal is to focus on yourself – not your speech – while making adjustments when necessary. This shift in perspective opens up a new vista, revealing the inner workings of stuttering and providing you with the keys to unlock your natural flow.

What I call 'control without controlling' is the state of unwavering certainty that you're in charge of your speech – not some elusive, external force that controls you at will. With this newfound sense of control, your fear and anxiety will begin to diminish, because you'll no longer feel like a victim of invisible forces that grip you and stifle your voice. Instead, you'll come to understand how stuttering works, break it down into manageable parts and take command of your own speech.

When you focus on stuttering, blaming it and seeing it as the root cause, you only create more tension, reinforcing the problem and delaying your progress towards freedom.

By adopting this new perspective, even when turbulence arises, you won't spiral into hopelessness or desperation. You'll recognize the true causes of your struggle, identify how you contribute to it through your own actions, and know how to self-correct. This prevents you from falling into the old cycle of blame, hopelessness, victimhood and self-criticism that once reinforced your stuttering. Instead, you'll break free from the blame game (and/or the shame game) and continue moving forward, preserving the progress you've made without being thrown back to square one.

I'll say it again: the key is to pull your attention away from the mechanics of speaking – and keep it away. The moment you focus on your speech, you return to the starting point, feeling stuck and overwhelmed by a seemingly insurmountable force called 'stuttering'.

Question 78:

I have several big presentations coming up for my internship and feel anxious about them. Despite doing this many times before, it never seems to get easier. How can I prepare effectively?

A: Please see the situation modelling practice mentioned in earlier responses.

'Mastery of self-control over your thoughts and feelings is your highest achievement!'

— Napoleon Hill

Question 79:

I just finished an online interview and, as expected, stuttered throughout. This was my first interview after graduation, and I feel terrible about it. Honestly, I wouldn't hire myself. I'm considering leaving white-collar jobs and focusing on other fields, like vocational work. What should I do? How can I change my situation?

A: '*As expected*' – there's your clue! We almost always manifest what we anticipate, rehearse or dwell on. Have you ever tried anticipating ease, composure and flow before an online interview? PWS are often experts at unconsciously manifesting verbal struggles. Your questions, like many others, illustrate this perfectly. You create vivid mental movies of these struggles, sometimes imagining them in great detail for days or even weeks before the actual event. If you anticipate failure, what else could you possibly expect to experience? Isn't this a form of self-imposed terror, rehearsing hardship instead of success?

'*I wouldn't hire myself*' – here's another key insight. This statement reveals a lack of self-love, and low self-esteem. If you don't believe in your own value, how can you expect potential employers to see it? Instead of contemplating leaving white-collar jobs because of anticipated difficulties, consider transforming the relationship you have with yourself. What if you began rehearsing success instead of failure? Address the underlying beliefs and narratives holding you back as soon as possible. When you build a foundation of self-compassion and belief in your worth, it will radiate outward. You'll find yourself not only speaking with greater confidence but also feeling more assured and comfortable in your own skin. This shift will undoubtedly enhance your chances of landing the job you truly desire.

Your current situation can change rapidly once you challenge and replace those limiting beliefs, attitudes and thought patterns that no longer serve you. Don't lower your standards; instead, elevate your mindset.

At your young age – just beginning your professional journey – it's important to recognize that life is not a rough draft. Each moment matters, and once time passes, it's gone. Why not start creating the best version of your life right now? Don't wait for 'someday' to live fully. Begin today.

Question 80:

I have a job interview for my dream job next week and I'm freaking out. My blocks are severe, sometimes lasting 30 seconds, and the only thing that helps is humming or making a sound before speaking, which I don't want to do in front of a panel. I hate this. My last two jobs were through connections, so I didn't have to interview, and my last real interview over a year ago went terribly. Any advice?

A: To put it simply, you're causing yourself unnecessary distress and creating your own hell on Earth. It's so clear from your description, but is it clear to you? You say you 'freak out, hate it, fear it' – the language you use reveals your attitude right away. Do you really expect to experience anything other than what you're currently creating – blocking, fighting, struggling? What you're doing is preparing for failure, and by even putting it in writing, you're sending a message to your subconscious mind that this is what you want. It's paradoxical, but we almost always end up manifesting what we fear and detest.

If you want to have better experiences, you must change your thoughts and expectations. By doing so, you'll shift the trajectory of your experience from negative to positive, from struggle to success. Try something new – prime yourself for success, not failure. And if it doesn't work, you can always return to your old ways. But the truth is, it will work.

For more detailed answers and practical tips, please refer to the earlier questions.

Question 81:

How do you manage teaching or careers that require a lot of speaking without feeling uncomfortable about your stutter? I'm considering online teaching but am terrified of negative comments. This fear and sense of inferiority make me feel demotivated and avoid such jobs. How do you handle these feelings and succeed in speaking-intensive roles.

A: I used to teach English and Russian both offline and online. When the idea of becoming a tutor first crossed my mind, stuttering never entered the picture. My focus was always on what I wanted, not on what I didn't want. If you step into this with an expectation of failure and the belief that others will be negative, then perhaps it's best to hold off for now. These thoughts – and the feelings of inferiority they create – are almost guaranteed to lead to the outcome you fear. You're setting yourself up for failure. Don't clip your own wings. Don't gaslight yourself.

Instead, I suggest you start by doing the opposite of what you've been doing. Take the same steps, but in reverse. If you practise this approach deliberately and consistently, you'll almost immediately begin to notice shifts. You'll start to understand how to regulate your emotions more effectively.

Question 82:

For single people who stutter, what's it like to attend social events and meet new people?

A: Everybody gets nervous, whether they stutter or not, because social situations are emotional by nature, not logical. 'Feel the fear and do it anyway' was my guiding mantra from the very beginning of this journey. What will help you immensely is learning to shift your attitude towards social events, regulating your emotions and treating yourself with kindness and respect. Be on your side, regardless of external circumstances.

I always recommend approaching any social situation with a playful, game-like attitude. This way, you won't feel as anxious or rigid, and you won't be as attached to the outcome or any expectations you might place on yourself. Focus on having fun and enjoying the experience, no matter the result!

Don't aim for perfection. Instead, aim for participation and connection with others. Even if you feel awkward, foolish or uncomfortable – which is completely normal – acknowledge and accept those feelings as an essential part of the learning process. You're learning to become socially confident, and this is a skill that takes time to develop, so don't be disheartened. Go with the flow and, please, don't take yourself too seriously. I believe the worst thing a person can do is take themselves too seriously.

It's perfectly normal to feel nervous. Don't resist it – flow with it – and you'll soon notice how quickly it dissipates, giving you the space and freedom to enjoy your social experiences in any setting, whether it's dating, meeting new people or just enjoying a conversation.

My final tip: don't try to impress, access!

Question 83:

What's the best way to address your stutter in a job interview without hurting your chances of getting hired?

A: Address yourself and your mind first. Let stuttering take care of itself.

If you approach an interview with an anticipation of failure, constantly replaying scenarios in your mind, emotionally investing in them and reliving imagined outcomes, you're setting yourself up for disappointment. Instead, imagine that you've already failed, and make peace with it. Forgive yourself, feel the relief that comes from letting go, and walk into the interview in this state of acceptance. I can almost guarantee your experience will be entirely different. Why? Because when you reconcile with the possibility of failure and forgive yourself, you relax both mentally and physically. You're no longer attached to the outcome.

Attachment and expectation create tension and stress, and these are precisely what you want to avoid. Here's where the magic happens: when you're free from attachment, you create space for spontaneity and fun. Fun brings lightness, and lightness allows you to be your authentic self. When you feel good about yourself, you flow, and that's when you succeed – not just in interviews but in life.

To overcome your speech and social anxiety, you need to do things differently – completely the opposite of how you've been approaching them. Make this new mindset a consistent practice until it becomes your natural way of being. And to ease your mind even further, remind yourself that this is not your last opportunity. There are countless other jobs out there. Even if this one doesn't work out, be grateful for the experience and keep applying.

If you're wondering whether you should disclose that you stutter, the answer is simple: if it helps you feel more relaxed and calm, then absolutely, yes. Do whatever you need to feel comfortable and confident.

Holistic and alternative approaches

Question 84:

When I drink alcohol, I feel more relaxed about my stutter and speak more freely. It's interesting how we often stay silent about our speech impediment due to others' opinions. How can we overcome this fear and speak more openly, regardless of what others think?

A: Substances – including alcohol, which is psychoactive – alter or diminish our inner dialogue and self-perception, changing our state of being and, consequently, our experiences.

When you drink, you may 'relax', which suggests that your inner dialogue becomes more benevolent and trusting, creating the conditions for relaxation. In that moment, you trust yourself, stop over-controlling and let go. If you pay close attention, you'll notice even your physical body becomes softer, less rigid. Habitual negative thought patterns shift or are temporarily replaced by positive ones, granting you a fleeting sense of freedom from inhibitions and insecurities. The heaviness of habitual thinking lifts for a while, leading to a sudden improvement in flow and ease.

However, the most important factor is not what others think of you – it's what you think about yourself. Ultimately, we create our inner experiences; no one else does this for us. That's why self-criticism is so toxic and disabling. It erodes us from within, silencing our voice and stifling our confidence. No external judgment can ever be as debilitating or have as crippling an effect as the harsh words we direct at ourselves.

Of course, there are people for whom alcohol has the opposite effect, worsening their speech or behaviour. This often indicates an especially strong compulsion to control (i.e. inner resistance) – so powerful that it doesn't even ease under the influence of alcohol.

'My program is not about positive thinking; it's about creating a new state of being using the natural tools already available to you. Those fleeting moments of flow you've experienced were the result of that "fluid" emotional state. I can teach you how to make it last – and how to switch it on and off at will.'

— Olga Bednarski

Question 85:

How is it possible for a person to not stutter when singing or talking to themselves?

A: There are laws of speaking, often referred to as vocal laws. When singing, these laws must be respected, and it's very difficult to break them, which is why you don't stutter. Additionally, every song has a defined tonality, pitch and pace that must be followed. This creates a structure that prevents you from 'improvising', thus keeping you aligned with the vocal laws. I believe that the melody of a song also promotes a more natural, flow-enhancing breathing pattern.

However, there are exceptions. When inner resistance is high, when trust is lacking and when there's a strong compulsion to control one's speech, stuttering can occur – even while singing. These cases are rare, but I do come across them from time to time.

With speaking, it's easier to break vocal laws simply because there's no set structure to follow, leaving you free to 'improvise'. If you happen to be someone who has ingrained habits of control – such as suppressing emotions, holding your breath or tensing your body – stuttering becomes a natural by-product of these psycho-emotional and physical dynamics, even if you're not fully aware of them. As John Harrison puts it, 'To speak fluently, you must get out of your own way – stop controlling and start letting go, surrendering.'

Question 86:

What in your opinion is the most effective treatment of overcoming stuttering?

A: It's my wholehearted conviction that PWS need education, not medical treatment, elaborate theories or medication. Education helps to replace the 'old malfunctioning software' with 'new, healthier software,' which, in turn, reduces – and eventually eliminates – the fearful reactions to speaking and communication in general. It also nurtures a healthier relationship with yourself and others.

What happens is that a person begins to become more themselves, more authentic. Irrational fears, anxiety and the tendency to hold back will no longer have a place in your life once you let go of fallacious, conditioned beliefs and return to your true self. There's now documented evidence and research showing how, by changing thinking patterns and beliefs, people have been able to self-heal from conditions that were once deemed incurable, including neurological ailments like Parkinson's, and even cancer. Most, if not all, so-called neurological conditions are triggered by our environment and the way we learn to respond to events and people.

Question 87:

How can PWS change their mindset?

A: By changing the way you think (i.e. ideas, narratives, stories) and how you feel about everything, you can transform yourself into a person who is free from fear, anxiety and the resulting stuttering. If you currently live in fear or anxiety, it means you're often thinking fearful, poisonous, anxiety-provoking thoughts. This process takes time and practice – there are no magic pills – but you can absolutely begin this journey on your own.

You can find free mindset audios on my channel, which I recommend for daily use. With consistent practice over at least three months, you'll begin to feel the effects and notice a significant transformation.

Question 88:

Can cannabis help with stuttering?

A: Cannabis may temporarily suppress excessive mental activity, which is why some people report improvement in their speech. However, much like alcohol or any other mind-altering substances, this positive effect isn't universal. For many PWS (and not just them, of course), mental activity is so hyperactive – constantly trying to stay in control – that it doesn't slow down, even when under the influence of these substances. I was one of those people. Alcohol never helped me relax; in fact, for fear of losing control, I became even more controlling, which made me unbearable to myself and others.

This simple explanation reinforces the fact – not just an opinion – that stuttering is caused and perpetuated by an untrained mind and its full identification with the problem. Once people learn to master their minds, things improve tremendously. What you truly need to control is not your speech, but the excessive mental activity that keeps it at bay.

Overcoming limiting beliefs and fear

'Becoming free from stuttering – letting go of holding back – is like discovering you have wings and learning how to use them.'

— Olga Bednarski

Question 89:

Due to my stuttering, I feel useless. How can I break this cycle and help myself?

A: Fluency is not a guarantee of happiness, lasting joy or meaning in life.

You don't feel useless because of stuttering; you stutter (hold back) because you believe yourself to be useless. It seems to me that you're stuck in a place of negativity, struggling to see beyond 'the bad' or the stutter. But you become what you think and feel. The thoughts in your mind create your emotional state – feelings of uselessness – that colour your entire existence and shape your reality. You don't even have to believe it consciously; the law works for all of us, without exception. Your inner states, whether of anxiety, calm, kindness, etc., all have physical manifestations in your body.

If you truly want to break the cycle, you must urgently work on changing your relationship with yourself and your thoughts (your inner dialogue). What you think determines your reality. Sometimes, people use their problems as excuses not to change, and blame the world for their misfortunes. Others, however, take their struggles and use them as fuel to inspire and help millions of others – like Nick Vujicic, for example. He had every reason to feel useless, but he chose a different path. So, it seems that feeling useful is a choice.

Over the years, you've developed a rigid 'working theory', as Dr Gabor Maté calls it. This theory of who you are is limited by past experiences and others' opinions that you took at face value. It's subjective and irrational, but it affects your life in very real ways, including how you feel about yourself.

The good news is that you can change this theory. You can shift into a qualitatively different state of being and begin to create brighter, more fulfilling life experiences. Relationships with yourself, just like with others, aren't permanent; they can be worked on, improved and healed. Ultimately, it all starts with you and deciding what you want for yourself.

Life, in its essence, is neutral. All situations are neutral. It's our minds that attach meaning to them – good vs bad, for example. You can help yourself out of the feeling of uselessness by intentionally seeking reasons to feel useful and to derive meaning from every moment of your life. Make it your daily intention to find meaning and purpose in each day. When it comes to overcoming stuttering, there's an abundance of help available, and much of it is free. If you seek it, you'll find it, and by applying it, you'll start seeing results. My YouTube channel is one such resource, full of tips on where to begin.

To overcome feelings of uselessness, I recommend spending as much time as possible doing what you love – things you have full control over, like a hobby or sport. Or, like me, you might choose to challenge yourself by joining a speaking club, finding your sense of meaning and self-inspiration in the process.

Don't let fluency become the condition for your happiness. Fluency is an external condition and, like all external things, once they're attained, they quickly lose their shine and no longer fulfil us – like buying a new car, for example. Realistically, how long does that joy last? Two to three weeks?

Instead, intend to become your own source of meaning and usefulness. Whatever choice you make, remember this: all changes require action. Nothing changes unless you change.

Question 90:

What we truly need is the freedom to speak without fear of embarrassment or rejection. People must respect and understand us as we strive to understand them. Greater awareness of stuttering among those around us can make our journey to recovery smoother. People who stutter often feel anxious and afraid due to the fear of being judged. What's your view on this?

A: I understand your frustration – it's completely valid. However, the position you're holding is a very limiting one, and will only lead you to more frustration, anger and a sense of unfairness. You'll inevitably encounter more people who don't understand, discriminate or reject you. And you'll find yourself waiting for something that may never come, because, realistically, society doesn't prioritize the issues of a minority that makes up just 1 per cent of the world's population. And why should they? Do you know every affliction, mental or physical, that exists? I doubt it.

Even when you say that you 'strive to understand them', what I sense here is not understanding, but indifference – a self-centred preoccupation with your own problem. Your 'understanding' is conditional, as if you're bargaining: '*If I offer you my understanding, what will I get in return?*' True understanding is unconditional. When you strive to understand others, it's not to gain something from them. Understanding does not expect anything in return, at least in my view.

Secondly, you have placed a condition in front of you: '*Unless society accepts me, I cannot accept myself. I cannot be happy, feel good about myself, or find peace.*' This self-imposed condition for happiness creates a barrier – a wall that forever separates you from what you want. The goal of universal acceptance is unlikely to be achieved, and as long as you tie your self-worth to it, you'll remain stuck. This is a dead-end road, and now it's time to turn around and find another way.

What you're trying to do is bend external circumstances to suit you, to control something that's beyond your control. This rationalization is dangerous and will cost you dearly in emotional well-being and time.

What you do have control over, however, are your feelings, attitudes and the way you choose to relate to situations and people. This is the key to gaining greater awareness of how you unknowingly perpetuate your stuttering, and it will make your journey to recovery smoother and faster.

You have two choices: you can continue to demand and get frustrated over society's ignorance, or you can change your attitude towards it, understand your stuttering and expedite your progress. If you choose the latter, you'll forget that you ever needed societal acceptance, and you'll get on with your life. You can either get busy living or keep complaining about society and miss out on your life.

What I want you to know is this: you don't need anyone's permission or acceptance to feel good about yourself right now. The freedom to speak without fear of embarrassment or rejection must come from within you, not from external forces, people or society granting you permission to feel worthy.

PWS often feel anxious and afraid because they struggle with self-acceptance and self-judgment. As I've said before, everything external is merely a reflection of our beliefs and attitudes towards ourselves.

The day you truly accept yourself is the day the world begins to accept you. Self-acceptance grows from self-compassion and self-love.

You attract whatever you emanate. If you emanate resentment and anger, guess what? You'll attract the same from others. People will subconsciously pick up on that energy and reflect it back to you.

Answering the following questions honestly will help you develop greater self-awareness, foster self-acceptance, clear your path and expedite your recovery:

- How would you feel and speak if you knew you were already accepted?
- How would you feel and speak if you had your own unconditional support in any situation, regardless of speech performance?
- How would you feel and speak if you knew, for certain, that people were more concerned with their own issues than with how you speak?
- How would you feel and speak if you saw people as more than just judges of your speech?
- How would you feel and speak if you stopped measuring your worth and social acceptability based solely on your 'speaking performance' and decided you're already worthy, just the way you are?

- What if you became curious about getting to know yourself beyond speech and about others as well?
- What if you authorized yourself to feel happiness and embrace all the good things you want in your life, without waiting for some external condition to be met?
- What if you saw that there are no real obstacles in your way, and the only roadblocks are your conditioned mind (e.g. '*Unless society accepts me, I cannot accept myself, feel good about myself or be happy*')?

Even if you achieved the goal of universal acceptance of stuttering, the satisfaction would only last for a brief moment. Don't go to war with society. Instead, focus on changing your perspective and your relationship with yourself. The benefits of this shift will far exceed your expectations. But you're the one who must take the first step; I can't do it for you.

Be the change you wish to see in the world. Accept yourself.

And, lastly, ask yourself: when you blame society and others for your lack of self-acceptance – isn't it madness?

Question 91:

Do you believe that shyness can exacerbate stuttering, while developing a strong and influential voice can help manage it better?

A: Shyness and timidity are closely tied to the system of speech anxiety. When we feel shy, a natural impulse is to retreat from situations, to 'shrink' into ourselves, becoming smaller and less visible. This isn't just psychological. Science has shown that our emotions directly affect the biochemistry of our bodies, leading to physical sensations like throat tightness, chest constriction and tension in the vocal cords. These feelings are your resistance embodied and often manifest as the infamous 'knot in the throat', a tight chest or voices that sound shrill, high-pitched or mousy.

Vocal training, especially when paired with confidence-building exercises, emotional regulation and mindful practices, can work wonders in releasing accumulated stress and even healing emotional trauma. These practices help free your voice, allowing it to become fuller, stronger and truly powerful – a reflection of your inner transformation.

Our voices are deeply connected to our inner world. The sound of your voice subliminally communicates how you feel inside – your emotional state, your confidence and even unresolved burdens you may be carrying. As you shift your inner dynamics, let go of what no longer serves you, and raise your energy (spiritually speaking), your voice naturally evolves too.

Question 92:

I'm currently pregnant with my first child and wondering if anyone else has kids who stutter. My husband doesn't stutter, but I do, and it makes me nervous.

A: The best thing a pregnant woman can do for her future child is to remain calm and at peace with herself. Worry, fear and anxiety only invite unnecessary troubles. I speak from my perspective of a mother here.

By worrying, you're unconsciously punishing yourself, hoping that somehow you can prevent problems from arising and spare your child from harm. However, this strategy does the exact opposite; it actually attracts the very things you fear. It's almost as if, deep down, you're secretly inviting these challenges. Why else would you devote so much of your attention to them? Worrying as a way to prevent problems is a common but misguided phenomenon, and it's considered normal in an unconscious world. But let me tell you this: worrying is not the same as caring – it's the complete opposite.

If you've read this far in my book, you already know that stuttering is a learned behaviour, an adaptive response, and therefore not hereditary. However, your temperament and tendency to experience anxiety may be passed down. Yet, the 'anxious gene' only predisposes you to anxiety; it doesn't automatically produce it. It's the environment that triggers and activates the gene.

Anxious mothers often raise anxious children, as young humans rely on the emotional regulation and nervous systems of their caregivers to regulate their own internal states (as Gabor Maté explains in *The Myth of Normal*). It's a scientific fact that stress is transmitted to a child while they're still in the womb. The anxiety you've described stems from your own unaddressed issues and early life experiences. This pattern is likely to continue unless you confront your past hurts and heal those inner conflicts. As Gabor Maté says, 'It's enormous work to recover from our childhoods. It's incredibly worthwhile, but it's a lot of work. The gospel of genetic causation shields us from having to confront our hurts, leaving us all the more at their mercy.'

If you want to protect your child from following in your footsteps, begin by exploring the hidden corners of yourself and decluttering your mind and heart. Additionally, arm yourself with knowledge about child psychology and development.

Personal growth and transformation

'Don't believe everything your mind tells you. Challenge and vet everything to dissolve the delusion.'

— Olga Bednarski, author of *The Anatomy of Stuttering*

Question 93:

It's painful to be held back by an impediment, wishing to be different, to not be on the sidelines and to feel fulfilled instead of empty. I long to express my thoughts and to be understood. How can I overcome my impediment and remove its psychological shackles?

A: There's nothing tangible or physical holding you back. What keeps you sidelined is the extent to which your mind identifies with your impediment – defining you as if you *are* it. When you see yourself solely through the lens of your stuttering, it drains life of its vibrancy and leaves you feeling empty.

Breaking free from these psychological shackles begins with understanding a vital truth: You are not your stuttering. It's merely a surface-level symptom trying to convince you otherwise. The second step is to give yourself permission to envision a different version of yourself. Imagine the person you would like to be without stuttering. How would that person feel, act, respond, behave and even carry themselves? Visualize this version of you in vivid detail – someone who no longer feels held back. As you dwell on this image, you begin to loosen the bonds of your old self-perception and start embracing this new, desired version of yourself.

This shift in perspective is challenging for many, especially for those who have never considered themselves as anything other than a person who stutters. That mindset can feel like a self-fulfilling prophecy, but it can absolutely be reversed. You don't have to live by the rule: 'Once a stutterer, always a stutterer.' Dare to exclude yourself from that narrative as well as from statistics and walk in a new direction – one where different actions lead to results you may not have even dreamed possible.

It's important to note, however, that action is key. Nobody can take those steps for you. The doing part is critical. But as you begin, you'll find it becomes easier and even enjoyable when you have a clear vision of the steps you need to take and the person you're becoming.

True freedom of expression – emotional emancipation – is not only possible but comes as a natural bonus of this inner work.

Question 94:

I find that depression and lack of confidence worsen my stuttering. When I feel good and am mentally sharp, I can speak much faster. Why does this happen?

A: Your question contains the answer. As your state of consciousness (your way of being) and how you feel about yourself shift, so too does your speech.

Depressive thoughts and the moods they bring tend to pull your mind inward (i.e. into unconsciousness, a trance-like slumber), dwelling on negativity and disconnecting you from the present moment. This 'falling asleep' or becoming unconscious often leads to becoming lost in mental projections and overwhelming ruminations, leaving you unable to notice what's truly happening around you. To break free from this unconscious state, reconnect with the present moment. Refer to my previous suggestions for simple and effective ways to do this.

When you become 'mentally sharp', your alertness and presence intensify. Your state of consciousness elevates – you rise above thought, as Zen masters and many spiritual teachers describe. In this state of sharpness and awareness, you're grounded and in control of your mind, which no longer interferes. Consequently, verbal struggles seem to vanish. How remarkable, isn't it? If stuttering were purely a genetic disorder, would such 'magic healings' or remissions occur? Surely not. If we must call stuttering a disorder, it's nothing more than a disorder of the untrained, restless mind.

When you inhabit the present moment, your thoughts naturally become more positive and affirming, unlike the unconscious state dominated by depressive patterns. Falling back into unconsciousness allows these default programs – like stuttering – to take over. The present moment truly is your moment of power. Hold on to it and cultivate the ability to return to it at will.

Here's a simple practice to help you reconnect: fully inhabit your body by focusing on the inner sensations within. Pay attention to what you might call the 'inner space' of your body and keep your awareness there. Just try it! Your body always exists in the now, and by reconnecting with it you anchor yourself in the present moment. This helps cultivate the mental sharpness you already know and can extend its presence in your life.

Also, begin observing your mind to identify what shifts it into this sharp state. Practise re-creating this mental clarity on demand. As you learn to master your mind, your stutter loses its grip. Remember, mastery of self-control over your thoughts and feelings is one of life's highest achievements.

Miscellaneous and unique perspectives

Question 95:

Has anyone else noticed that the climate crisis affects their speech and stuttering? I find that anxiety about the climate sometimes impacts my speech, causing me to stutter or shut down. Do others have similar experiences or thoughts?

A: The external climate does matter, of course. But when it comes to our feelings and state of being, it's our *internal weather* that matters most. While we have no direct control over the global climate crisis – and worrying endlessly about it can feel overwhelming and irrational – we *do* have direct control over our thoughts, emotions and how we choose to navigate our inner world.

If you truly wish to contribute to positive change on this planet, including how we treat nature and use resources, the wisest place to start is within yourself. By nurturing and healing your individual inner world, you become a part of the greater transformation.

Ultimately, I believe it's our collective inner worlds and shared consciousness that shape our behaviours, our actions and how we treat the Earth.

Question 96:

I took a karate class for fun and exercise. My speech greatly improved. Why?

A: As always, everything is simple. Physical activity helps reconnect you with your body and sends a signal to your brain that you're safe, aligning with the principles of mind-body connection. By engaging in physical activity, you move out of your head and into your body, becoming more deeply present in the moment. This shift naturally leads to improvement. Dancing, running or even gardening – if practised regularly – can have the same effect. And as an added bonus, you'll be in great shape, too.

'Suffering (and arrogance) comes from ignorance.'

— Olga Bednarski

Question 97:

I believe many problems stem from uneducated and backward societies. I'm working on acceptance and feel less depressed, but

people still interfere in my personal issues and judge. Recently, I was negatively judged, which made me very sad. I've never harmed others, so why do they hurt me? Have you experienced something similar, and how do you handle it?

A: Ignorance is the root of much human suffering. In other words, ignorance is a state of unconsciousness – a deep sleep we mistakenly call life. Sadly, unconsciousness remains the reality for the majority of people.

Your suffering comes from seeing yourself through the eyes of others and identifying with whatever negative things you hear about yourself. The truth is, the fact that people may speak negatively about you doesn't diminish your worth in any way. However, if you engage in negative self-talk and let the opinions of others define who you are, then that's where the true problem lies. People talking about us may sting, but it's the way we criticize ourselves from within that can tear us apart.

I sense that you may also be living from a victim mentality, which makes you more susceptible to criticism and negativity from others. Victimhood is like an open wound; it naturally attracts more hurt. I urge you to address this as a priority. Once you break free from the mindset of being a helpless victim, your relationships with others will begin to improve almost immediately.

I've been there too – I used to live in the role of the victim, and it was hell. I waited for others to love me, begged for their affection, but nothing changed. One day, I had enough. I stopped waiting for others to give me what I wanted and instead learned to give it all to myself. That's when things began to change, and they changed rapidly.

Question 98:

If there was a magic pill for stuttering, would you take it? If not, why not?

A: No, I wouldn't take a magic pill because it would cut short the beautiful and transformative journey of self-discovery.

Taking a magic pill is like winning the lottery. You might suddenly have the money, but with the same mindset of scarcity, you wouldn't know how to handle it. You might spend recklessly and end up losing it all, potentially landing in even greater debt than before. The same principle applies to stuttering. Freedom, while desirable, can also be intimidating!

Many PWS believe that fear of stuttering is their only obstacle and that once it's gone they'll immediately feel free and unconditionally happy. However, even if you achieve fluency, you may soon find yourself dealing with the same frustrations, resentments or feelings of sadness you had before – or even worse. Freedom brings its own set of challenges: new responsibilities, social pressures and expectations that inevitably change the pace and nature of your life.

True freedom requires readiness – a preparation period during which you cultivate a fluency mindset, learn to sustain it and grow comfortable with it. That's why I recommend approaching this journey step by step, allowing yourself time to adapt and feel at home with your progress. This gradual approach prevents overwhelm, resistance or discomfort and helps you avoid falling back into old habits.

Achieving fluency through a 'quick fix' like a magic pill might bring an initial wave of euphoria, but it could quickly give way to discomfort or even fear – fear of losing that fluency. This fear, as I've seen in many I work with, creates emotional and physical tension, leading to self-sabotage, doubt and eventually a return to the familiar yet limiting state of holding back.

There's more to overcoming stuttering than meets the ear. It's not just about speech – it's about transforming an entire mindset, personality traits, deeply entrenched beliefs, attitudes, habits and, most importantly, cultivating self-love and acceptance. These elements, no matter how effective the method or optimistic the outlook, can't be shifted overnight. It takes time to let go of the old 'stuttering self' and fully embrace the new fluent, free self. As the saying goes: 'Go slow to go far.'

Yes, there are miraculous stories of people healing from stuttering instantly, and while these cases, like that of Paul Stamets, are inspiring, they're rare and extreme exceptions.

'Nothing really matters except for inner peace, stillness, and peaceful joy. Whether others validate you or not – whether they say the words you long to hear – it won't make a lasting difference. The only true fulfilment, joy, and sense of control come from you accepting, embracing, and appreciating yourself. Only you can give it to yourself, and you can do it right now. It's just one conscious decision away.'

— Olga Bednarski, author of *The Anatomy of Stuttering*

Question 99:

Can you comment on suicidal ideation amongst stutterers?

A: People are often driven to suicidal thoughts by undisciplined minds – what we might call a 'monkey mind' – rather than external circumstances. Even if those situations seem overwhelming, unsolvable or dramatic, the truth is that dying cannot solve any problems. Only living – truly living, with intention and presence – can.

It's the mind that magnifies challenges and wraps them in a thick veil of illusion, creating what we call personal drama. What we perceive as problems are simply situations to be addressed and resolved. Through drama, undisciplined minds create disconnection from ourselves, trapping us in what feels like solitary confinement – a state we call 'living in the head' When this disconnection, which is essentially a separation from our spiritual essence, becomes too intense, it can push a person to the brink. Suicide, in this context, can be seen metaphorically as an attempt to return to oneself, to reconnect with the source.

It always saddens me deeply to witness this, because life itself is the ultimate gift. We're meant to live, to learn, to grow and to find happiness. I believe that premature death can often be prevented by helping people – especially those who stutter, but really anyone – understand themselves beyond their struggles. By learning how to self-regulate emotions and build a healthy relationship with themselves, with others and with the world, we can break free from the cycle of suffering.

Unconsciousness and ignorance are at the root of much of this pain. Once you truly understand who you are, how to live and how to embrace life with all its challenges, thoughts of ending your life will no longer hold any sway.

Question 100:

Why happens once anxiety and stuttering cease? Will I become unconditionally happy?

A: What remains when the illusion fades? Another illusion often arrives, ready to take its place. Our minds have a tendency to create problems or tasks – what I like to call 'missions' – as in my case. Fluency, just like stuttering, is an external thing, and thus it can be superficial. After the initial wave of freedom and euphoria, things will eventually settle into a natural rhythm, becoming part of your routine. It's similar to buying a new car – exciting at first, but after a few weeks or maybe a month that excitement fades.

Unconditional happiness, true joy, comes from emotional independence – from relying on nothing external. It's this peace and stillness that give birth to unwavering happiness.

No matter what you decide to do after overcoming stuttering or achieving fluency, I encourage you to have a bigger vision for your life. I hope you find a sense of purpose that brings deep meaning and fosters further positive change, beyond the external circumstances.

Question 101:

Is there scientific evidence of your approach working?

A: Give it a try, and you'll be the proof. I also invite you to read my first, research-based book on the subject, *The Anatomy of Stuttering* (2022).

'Don't swim with the current, or against it; swim where you need to go.'

— Eastern proverb

A Word on Support Groups for PWS

Do not let the well-meaning intentions of others hold you back from pursuing the life you dream of. In your journey towards freedom from limitations (speech anxiety) and true fulfilment, trust yourself above all else. Develop intellectual self-reliance (or intellectual self-defence) – it's your greatest ally.

I wholeheartedly support the idea of building communities where people can share their experiences without judgment, find encouragement and avoid the loneliness that often accompanies challenges. These spaces can offer much-needed comfort, understanding and connection. However, the safety and warmth of support groups can sometimes become stifling. They may limit personal growth, discourage deeper inquiry and block exposure to new perspectives.

One of the risks of such groups is that they can unintentionally reinforce the identity of 'stutterer', making it harder to see yourself beyond that label. These environments often attract speech pathologists or others who, despite good intentions, might perpetuate the narrative that stuttering is an immutable part of who you are. Even when groups aim to foster positivity with messages like 'you're not your stuttering', they sometimes contradict themselves by subtly suggesting that stuttering is unchangeable. The ego, once it identifies with something – such as stuttering – holds on to it tightly, resisting any challenge to that identity.

Ask yourself: would you rather cling to the comfort of such a group and remain in that identity, or take the risk of stepping outside that safety net to reclaim a fuller, freer sense of self?

Unfortunately, many support groups are insular and perpetuate a sense of victimhood under the guise of 'acceptance'. They encourage members to settle for the status quo rather than empowering them to rise above their predicament. This was my experience – if you don't support their narrative and identify as a victim, they simply don't know what to do with you. If staying in a victim role is a requirement for remaining in a group, then it's worth reflecting on what you truly want in life.

Remaining in the victim role may feel like a safe and cushy option, but it often involves subtle coercion to accept suffering as inevitable. Some groups and their organizers position themselves as the authority, offering advice and taking charge of members' lives. While this may come from a place of care, it can also prevent genuine empowerment and growth, which is concerning and, at times, even harmful.

The choice to join a group or not is entirely yours – but make it an informed one. Be discerning. Think for yourself. Do not let well-meaning but limiting narratives cloud your judgment or shield you from the potential for positive change. True support fosters growth, curiosity and self-discovery.

If you find a method or perspective that resonates deeply with you, pursue it wholeheartedly. Do not let others discourage you. Even if it doesn't lead to the outcome you hope for, you'll know you tried – and that in itself is freeing. I love how Paul Brocklehurst beautifully expresses it: '*Disillusionment is the path to enlightenment.*' On the other hand, if you feel your desire for change is met with resistance, discouragement or dismissal from your support group, it might be time to reconsider your membership.

Ultimately, your life is yours alone. You are your own authority. Choose support groups and people that support your growth, not ones that encourage helplessness or amplify victimhood.

About the Author

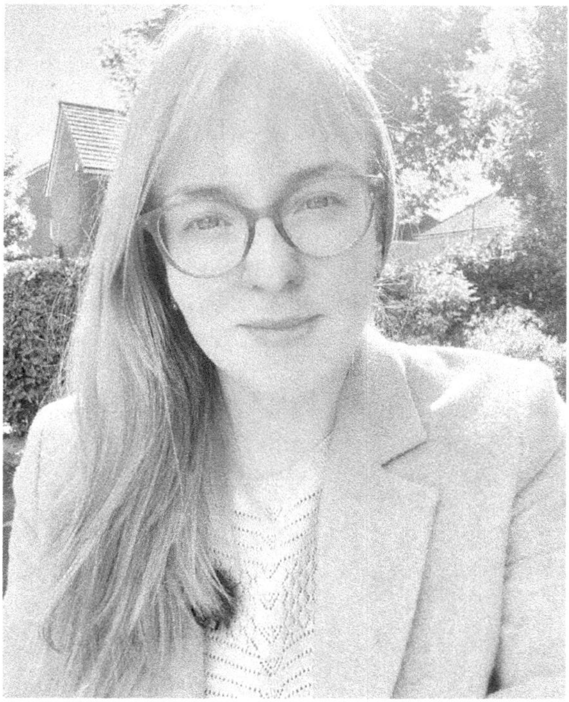

Olga Bednarski (BA Hons, MSc Psych.) is a dedicated stuttering expert and coach whose work is profoundly shaped by her personal journey of overcoming stuttering after living with it for over 18 years. Her approach, which diverges from traditional speech therapy, focuses on addressing the emotional and psychological roots of stuttering, such as anxiety and self-perception issues. Olga believes these aspects are often overlooked in conventional methods. Her philosophy emphasizes the power of awareness as a tool for mastering emotional self-regulation, dissolving fear, reducing hesitation and fostering quiet confidence and calm in social interactions.

Olga's expertise stems not only from extensive study and in-depth research but also from her lived experience. This combination forms the foundation of her unique approach. Her comprehensive research among individuals affected by speech anxiety led to the publication of her first book, *The Anatomy of Stuttering*, in 2022. With a first-hand understanding of stuttering, Olga provides insights and practical tools that go beyond theoretical frameworks, offering a real-world perspective grounded in personal transformation.

While not an accredited speech pathologist, Olga possesses a depth of knowledge and experience in the field of stuttering that surpasses many traditional practitioners, particularly as stuttering is a highly specialized niche within speech therapy. Her lived experience makes her a true case study, offering practical and empathetic solutions that resonate with those who stutter.

Olga is a passionate advocate for education that explores the deeper dimensions of stuttering and speech anxiety. She empowers individuals to overcome fear, embrace self-love and regain control over their speech, ultimately enhancing their quality of life. Through her work, Olga provides not only strategies but also inspiration and hope to others on similar journeys.

Additionally, Olga runs a dedicated YouTube channel, 'Stop Stuttering with Olga', where she shares guidance, fluency mindset audios and video lessons specifically for adults who stutter.

To learn more about Olga's work, coaching services, books and video products, visit: www.stopmystutter.com and www.olgabednarski.org

The Mission: Wholistic Wellness Company

Education is your medication: Education is your salvation

As a stuttering expert, my main mission is stuttering education. I strongly believe that PWS don't need magic pills, quick fixes or an overwhelming pile of elaborate theories with terminology that only confuse and mislead them. What's urgently needed is the right education – education that fosters awareness of deeper aspects of yourself beyond superficial symptoms and struggles, thus addressing the problem at its core origin.

Awareness delivered via education guides to individual wholeness and freedom; unawareness creates challenges and suffering that could have been easily avoided if only one knew and knew how. The right education provides understanding as to how PWS create struggle and contribute to anxiety, and it gives access to alternatives options of thinking, feeling, reacting and behaviours, thus opening the doors to novel, previously believed inaccessible, experiences of ease, lightness, enjoyment and composure in social situations.

I'm looking to establish a Holistic Wellness educational organization that, by means of various methods and practices, aims to help individuals with various mental health issues (not just speech anxiety) via development and cultivation of the exact set of personal qualities and skills that will greatly assist in reaching self-awareness on deeper level, enable understanding of the true root causes of their struggles and suffering and an ability to alleviate it and cease it. To awaken and empower individuals to their inner power to take charge and to change, regardless of their current mental state and life situation.

Opening the doors to positive new actions and change across all domains of life.

The Organization: Wholistic Wellness Company

Empowering individuals through awareness and education

The mission

I aim to transform lives through education that fosters self-awareness, authenticity, addressing the root causes of personal struggles and challenges, particularly for individuals who stutter or face speech anxiety. My goal is to empower people with the tools, insights and strategies necessary to cultivate inner awareness, break free (transcend) from fear and hesitation and unlock their full potential in communication and beyond.

The philosophy

I strongly believe that PWS don't need magic pills, quick fixes or overly complicated theories filled with confusing jargon. Instead, what they truly need is the right education – education that helps them explore the deeper aspects of their experiences, address the core origins of their struggles and replace them with ease, confidence and composure in social situations.

I focus on creating awareness, as it guides to freedom. Lack of awareness perpetuates unnecessary suffering and challenges that could easily be avoided with the right knowledge and skills. By showing people how they unconsciously create and contribute to their anxiety and offering alternative perspectives and behaviours, I aim to open doors to transformative experiences of lightness, enjoyment and empowerment.

The vision

I'm working to establish a Holistic Wellness educational organization to support individuals facing mental health challenges, including but not limited to speech anxiety. Through various methods and practices, I aim to help people develop greater self-awareness, uncover the true root causes of their struggles, and acquire the personal qualities and skills necessary to overcome them independently, without lifelong reliance on therapy.

My vision is to awaken and empower individuals to recognize their inner strength, take charge of their lives and embrace meaningful change – no matter their current mental state or life situation. By providing practical tools and guidance, I strive to facilitate personal transformation across all areas of life.

Ultimately, I aim to help individuals live with greater ease, freedom, and joy, making positive change not only possible but inevitable.

If you resonate with my work and feel you can contribute, I look forward to hearing from you and learning all about your ideas. Together, through our collective efforts, we can make the education of anxiety a transformative reality for many people sooner.

Epilogue

As I'm finalising this book, I'm standing on the shore of the Mediterranean Sea at Torre de Benagalbon, Spain watching the sun set. The insight crosses my mind – there was never anything wrong with me, there was not any problem, ever. The only problem was that I was fooled into believing that there was something terribly wrong with me. It's this belief that caused so much anguish, tears, pain, sleepless nights, hinderance and striving to fix that '*something that was wrong*', which could have been easily avoided, if only I realized this earlier.

I believe there was never anything wrong with you, too, my reader. All was and is always well. Now you must live according to this simple yet deeply profound realization. Remind yourself of it every day. Let it guide your thoughts, attitudes, reactions, behaviours and choices. Until it becomes automatic and effortless. Until it becomes your everyday experience and reality.

Upcoming Books and Projects

The Anatomy of Stuttering and Freedom: The Manual of Dissolution

Introducing *The Anatomy of Stuttering: The Manual of Dissolution* – a practical and empowering guide designed to help you navigate the path to freedom from anxiety while ensuring your hard-earned progress remains secure and lasting.

This instructional manual provides a clear, actionable plan tailored to your unique starting point, no matter the current severity of your speech anxiety. Filled with graphic visuals and step-by-step instructions, it's crafted to guide, inspire and keep you focused on your ultimate goal. Think of it as a trusted companion throughout your journey of personal transformation – offering encouragement, clarity and a steady sense of hope, even in turbulent times.

The guide emphasizes simplicity and practicality, featuring concise explanations paired with visual representations of the recovery process. Each step is thoughtfully laid out in an approachable manner to help you cultivate composure, trust and a sense of lightness, making freedom from anxiety an achievable, lived reality.

Inside, you'll find a transformative, step-by-step plan to:

- Manage and reduce anxiety.
- Prepare for various real-life situations.
- Develop emotional self-regulation practices.

These tools, and more, are designed to support you in creating lasting change.

The book also includes graphically illustrated insights into the mechanisms of stuttering, alongside practical approaches to mitigating or dissolving it – all without the need for constant reliance on a professional therapist or coach.

This manual will become your essential companion for several months, helping you make sense of your experience, uncover the subtle mechanisms underlying stuttering and cross over to a place of newfound freedom. Here, you'll learn how to masterfully navigate anxiety, maintain your results for a lifetime and embrace your fullest potential.

The Therapist in a Pocket ©: Self-Coaching Cards for People Who Stutter

Introducing a ground-breaking card set designed to revolutionize coaching and take self-help to the next level. These cards emphasize independence and the empowering idea that, equipped with the right tools, everyone can become their own unique guide and coach.

This is not your ordinary collection of positive-thinking reminders. These self-coaching cards are a powerful, transformative tool carefully crafted to spark profound change across multiple areas of your life. Their primary goal, however, is to help you achieve freedom from speech anxiety, cultivate a sense of flow and composure in interactions and maintain it for life. The result? Fluency that becomes a consistent, natural part of your daily experience – not an occasional accident.

Picture this: you're waiting in line for a job interview, preparing for a presentation or dreading a phone call. These self-coaching cards are your go-to resource, offering the advice, support and reassurance you need – right when and where you need it, literally in your pocket.

Each card is thoughtfully designed to guide you in:

- Self-regulating anxiety.
- Mitigating mental and physical resistance.
- Reducing tension.
- Developing and sustaining the mindset and emotional state conducive to natural, confident speech.
- Making new, more efficient choices in various situations.

With their help, you'll align your inner state with the outcomes you intend to achieve, fostering ease and flow in even the most challenging situations.

Consistent use of the cards is highly encouraged to maximize and expedite your progress. Over time, as you absorb and internalize their guidance, you'll find that coaching no longer comes from the cards themselves. Instead, the wisdom and encouragement will naturally arise from within you – empowering you to become your own coach, guide and source of support.

Also, see *The Anatomy of Stuttering* (2022)

Discover a ground-breaking alternative approach to freeing your voice with *The Anatomy of Stuttering*, the first book by Olga Bednarski, published in 2022 after years of dedicated research and practical experimentation.

This untraditional and insightful work offers a detailed, academically grounded exploration of speech anxiety – its mechanisms, how it manifests and, most importantly, how to strategically approach its dissolution. Far from being purely theoretical, the book integrates candid, illustrative accounts from individuals who stutter across the globe, making it relatable and deeply human.

The Anatomy of Stuttering serves as an excellent starting point for anyone seeking to understand speech anxiety and stuttering in depth. It dives into the intricate web of concepts and contributing factors that reinforce stuttering, presenting a well-rounded and research-backed perspective.

However, if you're ready to take your recovery to the next level and desire a more practical, hands-on approach to overcoming stuttering, I encourage you to explore my book *Speech Anxiety & Stuttering: 101 Questions and Answers About Stuttering in Adults* (2024).

This research-based book is also an invaluable resource for open-minded speech pathologists and researchers in the field of speech disorders and communication, offering fresh insights and tools to better understand and support individuals on their journey to fluent self-expression.

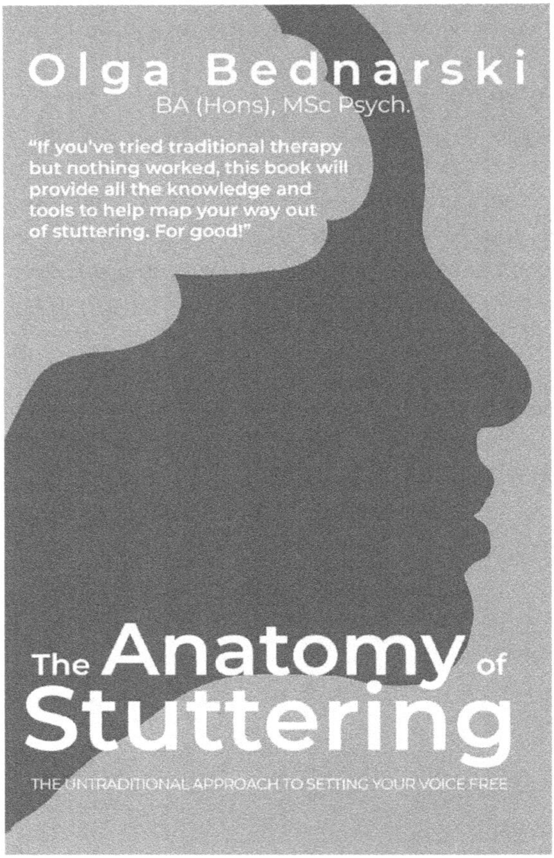

Olga's YouTube channel and further support

Visit my YouTube channel, **Stop Stuttering with Olga**, for more valuable insights, practical tips and self-help tools – such as daily mindset audios designed to support and empower you on your journey to freedom from anxiety. These resources will help you stay motivated, build confidence and firmly set you on the path of lasting transformation.

The end.

The end to suffering, the end to stuttering.

Books of Interest and Resources

Bednarski, O. (2022). *The Anatomy of Stuttering*. Wholistic Wellness Company.

Brocklehurst, P. (2016). *The Perfect Stutter*. Independent Publishing.

Harrison, J. *Redefining Stuttering: What the Struggle to Speak Is Really All About.* National Stuttering Association.

Maté, G., & Maté, D. (2022). *The Myth of Normal: Trauma, Illness, and Healing in a Toxic Culture*. Avery.

Hawkins, D. R. (2001). *The Eye of the I: From Which Nothing is Hidden*. Veritas Publishing.

FreeStutteringBooks.com is a website dedicated to providing free e-books and resources for individuals who stutter, as well as for parents, teachers and speech-language pathologists. Additionally, it includes French translations of selected materials, TED Talks and other relevant videos.

www.ingramcontent.com/pod-product-compliance
Lightning Source LLC
LaVergne TN
LVHW022220200926
848481LV00006B/2044
* 9 7 8 1 0 6 8 1 5 2 0 3 0 *